The Ethics of Human Gene Therapy

The Ethics of Human Gene Therapy

LeROY WALTERS
JULIE GAGE PALMER

*With illustrations by
Natalie C. Johnson*

New York   Oxford
OXFORD UNIVERSITY PRESS
1997

Oxford University Press

Oxford   New York
Athens   Auckland   Bangkok
Bombay   Bogota   Buenos Aires
Calcutta   Cape Town   Dar es Salaam   Delhi
Florence   Hong Kong   Istanbul   Karachi
Kuala Lumpur   Madras   Madrid   Melbourne
Mexico City   Nairobi   Paris   Singapore
Taipei   Tokyo   Toronto

and associated companies in

Berlin   Ibadan

Copyright © 1997 by Oxford University Press

Published by Oxford University Press, Inc.
198 Madison Avenue, New York, New York 10016

Oxford is a registered trademark of Oxford University Press

Library of Congress Cataloging-in -Publication Data
Walters, LeRoy.
The ethics of human gene therapy /
LeRoy Walters, Julie Gage Palmer.
p.   cm.   Includes index.
ISBN 0-19-505955-7
1. Gene therapy—Moral and ethical aspects.
I. Palmer, Julie Gage.
II. Title.
RB155.8.W35   1996   174'.25—dc20   96-33680

9 8 7 6 5 4 3 2 1

Printed in the United States of America
on acid-free paper

To Robert, David, and Sue,
and in memory of Jane
To Joseph, David, and John

Preface

This book has had a 10-year gestation period. It was initially suggested by Mr. William F. Curtis, then Editor at Oxford University Press. Mr. Curtis had seen a short commentary in *Nature* entitled "The Ethics of Human Gene Therapy," written by one of the authors. In a letter dated April 7, 1986, he asked whether a short book on this topic might not be "useful and instructive."

Soon after this invitation arrived, the two of us discovered that we were both deeply interested in the topic of gene therapy and that our fields of training provided complementary perspectives on the science and ethics of this promising technique. We therefore agreed to work together on a joint book. The research for and writing of this book have been a cooperative effort in every respect and at each stage. Neither of us would have attempted, or could have completed, this project on our own.

While we would like to have concluded our work several years ago, this is an appropriate moment for appraising the first stage of gene therapy research with human patients. Since September 1990, when the first patient was treated in an approved study, more than 100 additional gene therapy protocols have been written and submitted for approval. At the same time, however, we have the sense that in 1996 many researchers in the field are pausing to catch their breath. There are important scientific findings in a few studies, and intriguing hints of benefit in others. Yet, on the whole, the diseases that plague human beings have proven to be much more difficult to defeat than some researchers had anticipated. Thus, our book provides an overview of gene therapy at the end of its first phase. In our opinion, this phase will be followed by redoubled efforts and even more creative approaches to treating a broad spectrum of human maladies.

Both of us have experienced serious illness and premature death in our own families. In part for this reason we identify strongly with the patients who have participated in the early clinical trials of gene therapy, as well as with the researchers who have designed gene-therapy protocols in an effort to help them. We include in the Introduction to this book a brief memoir of David, the courageous young man from Houston who spent his entire life protected from the outside world by a plastic bubble. No family and no health care providers could have done more for a child than those around David did for him. Yet tragically, the new approaches to treatment that are helping other children with diseases like David's—including gene therapy—became available only after his death.

In the 10 years that we have been working on this book, both of us have received helpful suggestions, constructive criticism, and moral support from numerous colleagues, friends, and organizations. We run the risk of failing to acknowledge some of those who have assisted us if we mention names, but our debts of gratitude are so great that we cannot be content with general expressions of thanks.

JGP wishes to thank Noel Gage, Hilda Gage, and Jacqueline Gage for lifelong encouragement and support. In addition, she thanks the Harvard Department of Special Concentrations, Jonathan Beckwith, Rebecca Eisenberg, W. French Anderson, Judith Areen, the law firm of Hopkins & Sutter, Eric Juengst, Mark Siegler, John Lantos, Mary Mahowald, and the University of Chicago's MacLean Center for Clinical Medical Ethics for supporting and encouraging her study of gene therapy. JGP is grateful to Kathy Schlegelmilch for her cheerful, highly skilled secretarial assistance.

JGP would also like to thank LW for encouraging her interest in gene therapy, for generously providing her with the opportunity to work on this project, for his careful, intelligent comments on her drafts of sections of this book, and most of all, for many years of warm, supportive friendship. Sue Walters has also been a tireless champion of this work and a wonderful friend to Julie.

JGP owes her greatest debt of gratitude to her husband, John B. Palmer III, who supported her work on this book with emotional encouragement, financial sacrifices, research assistance, and many hours of excellent editing work.

LW would like to thank his colleagues at the Kennedy Institute of Ethics, Georgetown University, for their interest and encouragement during the entire time that this book was being written. These colleagues are Frances Abramson, Ariella Barrett, Tom Beauchamp, Laura Bishop, Gregory Cammett, Mary Carrington Coutts, Martina Darragh, Ruth Faden, Marc Favreau, Doris Goldstein, Moheba Hanif, John Collins Harvey, Kristen Heavener, Lucinda Fitch Huttlinger, Joy Kahn, Rihito Kimura, John Langan, Margaret Little, Pat McCarrick, Charles McCarthy, Irene McDonald, Kathy McMahon, Bill Mosqueda, Hannelore Ninomiya, Anita Nolen, Kier Olsen, Barbara Orlans, Cecily Orr, Edmund Pellegrino, Madison Powers, Warren Reich, Kathy Reynolds, Hans-Martin Sass, Carol Mason Spicer, Robert Veatch, Kevin Wildes, and Emily Wilson. These colleagues have been wonderful friends, as well as highly-competent professionals. The Philosophy Department at Georgetown University has also been very supportive, and especially the Department Chair, Wayne Davis. During the writing of this book, the members of the Recombinant DNA Advisory Committee (RAC) at the National Institutes of Health (NIH) and the RAC's Human Gene Therapy Subcommittee have been constant sources of intellectual stimulation and expert advice to LW. The committee and subcommittee have been supported with consummate professionalism by the NIH Office of Recombinant DNA Activities, especially Christine Ireland, Debbie Knorr, Becky Ann Lawson, and Nelson Wivel.

LW also acknowledges with gratitude a grant from the Joseph P. Kennedy, Jr. Foundation and its Executive Director, Mrs. Eunice Kennedy Shriver, that supported the early stages of his research. The National Science Foundation and the National Endowment for the Humanities also provided partial funding for the research on this book through grants RII-830987 and RII-8443766 ("Ethical Issues in Human Gene Therapy"). LW would also like to thank Georgetown University and the Kennedy Institute of Ethics for two sabbatical leaves during the writing of this book. The provision of an endowed chair by the Kennedy Foundation and his selection to fill the chair by President Leo J. O'Donovan, S.J., of Georgetown University have allowed LW to spend three months each summer in a delightful combination of rest and research.

LW is also grateful for the collaboration and insight of JGP throughout the entire process of writing this book. JGP's technical knowledge has helped us to avoid numerous pitfalls, and her perseverance has kept this joint project moving forward. She has also been an empathic friend during times of sadness and times of renewed hope.

Without the support and forbearance of his immediate family, LW would not even have attempted this work. His late wife Jane and two young children, David and Robert, were present and involved as LW's research on the book began. His wife Sue and two children who are now young adults have been both patient and understanding as the book has gone through the final stages of revision and production. LW's debt of gratitude to these four generous and caring people can never be repaid.

Both authors would like to thank several people who have read and commented on drafts of this work. They include Robert Cook-Deegan, Sharon Durfy, Martin Eglitis, Kevin FitzGerald, Michael Grodin, Eric Juengst, Brian Lindman, Stephen McCormack, Karen Peterson-Iyer, Jeffrey Rosenberg, and Kenneth Schaffner. Marc Farreau assisted in the preparation of the index.

Our work has been ably, and patiently, facilitated by Mr. Jeffrey W. House at Oxford University Press. Mr. House has tried to keep us on track and he has brought important new publications to our attention. We also wish to thank our anonymous but gifted copy editor and our Production Editor, Ms. Nancy Wolitzer, who has expertly turned our manuscript into well-designed pages. Our illustrator, Natalie Johnson, has been an active participant in this project for the past two years and has succeeded in translating our text into clear, striking images.

We have dedicated our book to our spouses and our children, without whose love and encouragement this work would never have come to completion.

Washington, D.C.   L. W.
Chicago, Illinois   J. G. P.
June 1996

Contents

Introduction

David was born at 7 A.M. on September 21, 1971. His older brother had died 10 months earlier of a rare genetic disorder called severe combined immune deficiency, or SCID, for short. This disease prevents both major parts of the immune system from functioning, thus leaving any child with SCID completely vulnerable to any bacteria or viruses in the environment. In fact, David's older brother had been afflicted with a series of infections that did not respond to the usual antibiotics. He had succumbed to pneumonia at the age of 7 months.[1]

Because of the possibility that David, too, would be afflicted with SCID, extraordinary precautions were taken at St. Luke's Episcopal Hospital in preparation for his birth. A special germ-free room was prepared for David's mother, and delivery-room physicians and nurses silently prepared for a caesarean delivery in an operating room where no speaking would be permitted in order to minimize the probability of infection. Ten seconds after his delivery, David was placed in a plastic isolator bubble. Later that day he was transferred to the Clinical Research Center at Texas Children's Center, which was next-door to St. Luke's.

For the next 2 weeks David remained in the isolator bubble while his caretakers performed laboratory tests to determine whether he too had severe combined immune deficiency. David's parents were at home when the doctors called and asked them to come in for a meeting. David's mother described the meeting.

Two doctors were waiting for us when we walked into David's room. We had spent so much time with them during the previous few months that we felt close to them and knew immediately by the pain on their faces that the news was bad. They told us that David did indeed have the same problem that had killed his older brother. If he was not continuously shielded from the everyday world, he, too, would die. Then they left us alone with our son.[2]

When David was 2 months old, he was allowed to go home for 4 days in the isolator bubble for the Thanksgiving holiday. A month later he was home for 2 weeks for the family's Christmas celebration. Shortly thereafter, David's family converted the living room of their home into a protected shelter for David. The largest module in the shelter was an 8 × 10 foot playroom with solid sides. A flexible plastic transport bubble was attached to one side of the playroom, and a supply bubble and a crib bubble were attached to a second side. Gloves built into the sides of the crib and transport bubbles allowed his parents to care for David without actually touching him. Filtered air was continuously pumped into the shelter.

David had a close relationship with his sister, Katherine, who was almost 4 years older than he. (Because David's type of SCID was sex-linked, that is, only affected males, his sister was free of the disease.) From the time when he first came home for Thanksgiving until her 13th birthday, Katherine insisted on sleeping in the living room next to David's transporter bubble. Closeness did not, however, preclude conflict. Periodically, David and Katherine's mother would have to intervene to break up a fight between the two siblings. On one occasion the brother and sister were using the built-in gloves to slam each other around, "much to David's delight."[3]

By the time he was 3 years old, it was clear that David was a gifted child. When he was old enough, he began attending school by speakerphone. His classes usually lasted from 8 A.M. until noon. Through the speakerphone David was able to converse with his teachers and fellow students. On occasion the other students and his teachers stopped by the house to help with homework. At other times David's class came to his home for special entertainment programs. David enjoyed using hand puppets, playing music on his recorder, and participating in spelling bees with the class. In his classwork David made straight A's. He especially enjoyed geography and mathematics.

When David was about 5, a kind of space suit was designed for him. The suit looked similar to the suits worn by NASA astronauts. With the aid of the suit David could explore other rooms of his home and even walk around outside for a short time. However, the air supply and batteries for the space suit only lasted for about 4 hours at a time. When David outgrew the first space suit, no second suit was ever built because of concerns about legal liability. According to David's mother, it was unclear "who would be responsible in case of accident while he was using it."[4]

Throughout his life David always looked forward to one day being liberated from his protective bubble. According to his mother,

We lived with the hope that some treatment or cure would be discovered to allow David to leave his bubble and lead a normal life. The possibility of that happening was a sustaining force for all of us, including my husband, David, and our daughter, Katherine, and David's attitude was heartening. He always felt that *when*, not *if*, he got out, everything would be all right. He never talked about *not* getting out.

• • •

From the time he was small, David talked about the kind of life he wanted when he left the bubble. Once, seeing his uncle sweeping the front porch, he called out, "When I get out of this bubble, I'm going to help do that." At other times he talked about being a fireman. I remember telling him jokingly that as a Catholic mother, I wanted him to go to Notre Dame and become a priest. Knowing something of the dedication and deprivation of the priesthood, he laughingly told me, "You can forget that."[5]

By the time David was 11, bone marrow transplantation techniques had improved to such an extent that David's family began to think seriously about the possibility of a transplant. During the summer of 1983 the family agreed on this step as the best and perhaps only hope for freeing David from his confinement to the bubble. Donor tests were performed, and David's sister, Katherine, proved to be the best matched donor. On October 21st, 1983, 1 month after David's 12th birthday, Katherine and her mother flew to Boston, where some of Katherine's bone marrow was harvested and treated so that it would not attack David's cells after the transplant. A few hours later, at Texas Children's Hospital in Houston, David received an infusion of his sister's bone marrow cells. Inside his bubble, David assisted the doctors by placing the needles for the infusion into his own veins.

The day of the infusion was followed by weeks of waiting and hoping that Katherine's bone marrow cells in David's body would begin to produce the enzyme that his own cells were lacking and allow his immune system to begin functioning for the first time. By mid-December there was still no evidence that the transplant had taken, and the family began to feel "twinges of apprehension."[6] David was allowed to go home for Christmas and gave his sister Katherine a special gift, a sapphire-and-diamond ring, as a token of his thanks to her for being his donor. On New Year's Day 1984, David routinely took his temperature and found that it was 99.5° F. The following day David was scheduled to return to the hospital. He mentioned his fever to the nurses, but they did not seem worried. However, within a few days David began to run fevers as high as 105° F. Medication could reduce the fever, but David had difficulty keeping food down and sometimes suffered from serious diarrhea. His doctors began worrying that he would become dehydrated and said that, if he needed intravenous fluids, he would have to come out of his protective bubble.

David's condition continued to deteriorate. On February 7th, 1984, he was gently removed from his bubble by his physician, Dr. William Shearer. Once outside, David was fascinated by the direct view he had of objects that he had previously been able to see through a thin sheet of plastic. Even though he was groggy from his illness, David "ran his fingertips over the furniture and lifesaving equipment."[7]

Despite the desperate measures being taken on his behalf, David's illness grew more severe. He began to vomit blood, and the intervals between his raging fevers grew shorter.

On February 22nd David seemed to sense that he was losing the battle for life. In the words of his mother,

> He told the doctor, "I'm tired. Why don't we just pull all the tubes out and let me go home?" By "home" I think he meant to say he knew he was dying, and a better place awaited him. Then he winked at the doctor.
> The tubes were taken out, as he had asked. He had been free of the bubble for 15 days. He was placed on a respirator to ease his breathing. Dr. Shearer gave him a sedative to ease his last hours.
>
> • • •
>
> We all stepped outside, and a few minutes later, at five minutes until 8 in the evening, the doctor came into the room and told us David had died.[8]

In May 1985, 14 months after David's death, Dr. William Shearer and his colleagues published a report in the *New England Journal of Medicine* in which they analyzed the cause of David's death. An autopsy performed on David's body and detailed laboratory studies revealed that David had contracted an Epstein-Barr virus infection from the bone marrow cells donated by his sister. The reason for David's abrupt clinical decline was now clear. In his sister's body, a normally-functioning immune system had been able to keep the Epstein-Barr virus in check. However, after David received the bone marrow transplant, including some cells infected with the Epstein-Barr virus, his severely compromised immune system was not able to control the virus. As a result, the virus attacked the few B cells (white blood cells that produce antibodies to infection) that were present in David's blood. The infected B cells began dividing rapidly and soon became malignant. The malignancy, called a B-cell lymphoma, quickly spread to all of David's major organs. It was this raging lymphoma that overwhelmed his body and caused his death.

Thanks to news stories published at the time of David's death and to the courage of his mother in helping to tell his story to the world, we know something of the struggle against disease that David and his family endured. We can only stand back in silence and in profound sadness as we reflect on the tremendous efforts undertaken by David, his parents, his sister, and the doctors and nurses who provided his care. Despite these heroic efforts, David died tragically at the age of 12.

It is because of the death of David and because of thousands of other untimely deaths of children and adults, most of whose names we do not even know, that the field of human gene therapy is important. Gene therapy is the attempt to cure or prevent disease at the most basic level—at the level of DNA and the genes that are composed of DNA. The diseases that are being targeted in gene therapy studies are not only inherited disorders like the SCID that afflicted David. Researchers have also designed studies that are exploring whether this new technique will be effective against various kinds of cancers and against AIDS.

   This book seeks to describe the science of gene therapy in terms that are accessible to laypeople and to examine the major ethical questions that are raised, and that are likely to be raised in the future, by human genetic intervention. The plan of our book is as follows. In Chapter 1, we provide a brief overview of DNA, genes, and cells and how they function in all organisms, including human beings. Chapter 2 discusses the kind of gene therapy that is currently being performed at numerous research centers around the world. This kind of gene therapy is similar in some respects to common treatments like blood transfusions, bone marrow transplants, and organ transplants. In Chapter 3, we consider gene therapy techniques that would aim to prevent disease not only in an individual patient but also in that patient's children and grandchildren. In other words, we explore the notion of preventing disease through changing genes in reproductive, or germ-line, cells. Chapter 4 moves away from the context of health care and medicine in the strict sense and asks: Can genetic techniques be used to enhance human capabilities? If so, *should* these techniques be used for this purpose? In the final chapter we examine how gene therapy has been handled as a public policy question since the late 1960s. This chapter will indicate how an open national review process has provided unprecedented public access to information on a new biomedical technology.

   Two important distinctions underlie our analysis in Chapters 2, 3, and 4. The first is the distinction between somatic and germ-line cells, which includes germ cells and germ cell precursors. This distinction is significant because, unlike somatic cell genetic alterations, germ line genetic alterations will likely be transmitted to future generations. The second distinction is less clear-cut. It is the distinction between the prevention, treatment, or cure of disease, on one the hand, and enhancement of human characteristics or capabilities, on the other. If gene therapy matures into a successful disease treatment, it is likely that the newly developed techniques for manipulating genes will be serviceable for "improvement" as well as treatment. The following matrix illustrates the four types of genetic intervention that follow from these two conceptual distinctions.

	Somatic	Germ Line
Prevention, treatment, or cure of disease	1	2
Enhancement of capabilities or characteristics	3	4

Each category of genetic intervention, 1 through 4, presents its own set of issues, which we will address in turn. Chapter 2 will be devoted to type 1 genetic intervention in somatic cells for the prevention, treatment, or cure of disease. Chapter 3 will address type 2, genetic intervention in germ line cells for the prevention, treatment, or cure of disease. Chapter 4 will focus on types 3 and 4, genetic intervention in somatic and germ cells, respectively, for the enhancement of human capabilities or characteristics.

Notes

1. The following account of David's life is based primarily on a two-part story published in *People Weekly* on October 29th and November 5th, 1984 (Carol Ann with Kent Demaret, "David's Story," *People Weekly*, October 29, 1984, pp. 120–124+, and "The Bubble Boy: Part II," November 5, pp. 107–108+). See also Larry Thompson, *Correcting the Code: Inventing the Genetic Cure for the Human Body* (New York: Simon and Schuster, 1994), pp. 15, 41–42.
2. "David's Story," October 29, 1984, p. 125.
3. Ibid., p. 141.
4. Ibid., p. 138.
5. "The Bubble Boy: Part II," *People Weekly*, November 5, 1984, p. 108.
6. Ibid., p. 120.
7. Ibid., p. 122.
8. Ibid., p. 127.

The Ethics of Human Gene Therapy

1

Genes: Function and Heredity

During the course of humankind's struggle to understand the mysteries of life, a theory emerged that explained how human traits were determined and inherited. Many people subscribed to this controversial *theory of preformation* in the late 1600s and for two centuries thereafter. According to this theory, human characteristics or traits passed from parent to child via homunculi, which were tiny worms present in human sperm. Preformation adherents believed these worms were preformed, miniature adults that simply enlarged during pregnancy.

Modern technology has uncovered a more flexible and more elegant explanation of the derivation and descent of human characteristics. The fundamental element of this explanation is a functional unit called a gene. Genes govern the incredibly diverse panoply of human traits, and genes are the purveyors of the efficient process by which these traits are mixed, matched, and passed from one generation to the next.

As our understanding of genes grows, so does our ability to manipulate them. This ability to manipulate the fundamental elements of human characteristics and heredity promises to spark some of the most important and difficult debates of human history. This book will attempt to explain how genes can be manipulated and to wrestle with some of the issues that arise therefrom. In order to begin, it is necessary to introduce genes, their structure, their function, and the role they play in heredity.

Genes

Every cell in a person's body contains a complete set of genetic information. Different genes are turned "on" and "off" in different cells and at different stages in development. Genes tell a cell how to behave, what proteins to produce, when to grow, when to stop growing, what shape to take, and more. Genes direct the various traits of each human being by controlling the differentiation of the billions of cells in each individual's body. Together, the total genetic information contained in a person's genes comprises a *genome*, a unique genetic blueprint for each person.[1]

A person's entire genome can be found inside each cell in the same central location. Although cells come in many different forms, most share the same basic structure. They have an outer envelope, or *membrane*, which encloses the substance called *cytoplasm*. The cytoplasm contains many specifically functioning structures called *organelles*, including *ribosomes*, where genetic information directs protein synthesis. The central organelle, the *nucleus*, is a sphere-like structure that contains the genes.[2]

When genes function normally, they form the foundation used by each cell in performing its functions at the appropriate time and place, so all the cells in a person's body act in concert, collectively forming the tissues with which we move, breathe, digest, and think. Like a musician in an orchestra plays certain notes at precisely the right moments, a functioning cell "plays" certain genes in just the right amounts at just the right times. Genes comprise intricate written instructions which cells heed in the same way musicians follow a musical score. The result is more complex and more eloquent than even the most complex symphony.

If all genes functioned normally, all human beings would be free of genetic disease. However, errors in the structure or function of genes are inevitable (and, in fact, necessary to the forward march of evolution).[3] Some errors may be so slight or insignificant that the result is hardly noticeable, like the effect on a symphony when one violinist in an orchestra accidentally plays one flat note. Other genetic errors may disrupt a vital function and thereby threaten life itself, like a symphony never begun. Many diseases fall between these extremes. A genetic disease may allow one who suffers from it to live, but may impair his or her ability to function, like a symphony played with the percussion section missing or with one clarinet continuously playing the same note, even when it is not supposed to play at all. As many potential disruptions of a symphony as one can imagine, there are more potential errors to be found in our genes.

Gene therapy is the attempt to treat diseases that result from these errors by adding new genes to cells or by substituting new genes for original malfunctioning genes. Rather than simply responding to disease symptoms, this therapeutic approach seeks to attack diseases at their root by altering the basic instructions that control how our cells function—the instructions provided by the genes. Even in situations where gene therapy cannot correct the malfunction in a type of cell, this new approach may confer new disease-fighting capabilities on cells. For example, genes introduced into human cells may be infused into patients in a procedure like a blood transfusion. Once inside the patient, these genetically modified cells can produce drugs that will help to counter the patient's disease. In other words, gene therapy can function as a new kind of drug-delivery system.

Gene Structure and Organization

Genes are comprised of deoxyribonucleic acid (DNA). DNA is a molecule that consists of two intertwined strands, wrapped around each other in helical fashion, like the stripes of a barbershop pole. Accordingly, when James Watson and Francis Crick discovered DNA's structure in 1953, they called it a *double helix*.

Each of the two DNA strands has a backbone located on the outside of the double helix. The backbone is composed of repeating compounds of phosphate and deoxyribose (a kind of sugar). On the inside of the DNA double helix, flat, ring-shaped molecules called *bases* are strung along the sugar-phosphate backbone. These bases contain carbon and nitrogen (Figure 1–1).

Each base is attached to a deoxyribose molecule which is attached to a phosphate group. The whole unit is called a *nucleotide* (Figure 1–2). The nucleotides are linked one to another along the backbone of each strand by regularly repeating chemical bonds, something like Lego pieces, each stuck in identical fashion to its neighbor.

Two classes of bases are found in DNA, the purines and the pyrimidines. There are in turn two purine bases: adenine (A) and guanine (G), and two pyrimidine bases: cytosine (C) and thymine (T). The bases, attached to the inside of the two helical backbones, face each other and pair up, forming hydrogen bonds between them. Because of their molecular structures, A can pair only with T, and G can pair only with C. The hydrogen bonds between these "base pairs" hold the two chains of the double helix together[4] (Figure 1-3).

Although all genes are made of DNA, not all DNA makes up genes. The bases are strung along in varying order along the double helix, sometimes constituting genetic information and sometimes not. Some base sequences serve as a kind of scaffolding that holds the double helix in secondary or tertiary structures. A single long strand of DNA will contain several genes, many structural sequences, and plenty of sequences whose functions are unknown. Whatever the sequence may be on one strand, the opposing, or *complementary*, strand has corresponding bases. For example, if the sequence of bases along one strand is AACGTTA, the sequence along the other strand will be TTGCAAT. Genes can be found on both strands.

Only a small fraction (between 1/20th and 1/35th) of the 3 billion base pairs of human DNA represents genes.[5] Researchers estimate that there are between 50,000 and 100,000 human genes; 80,000 genes seems to be the most likely estimate.[6]

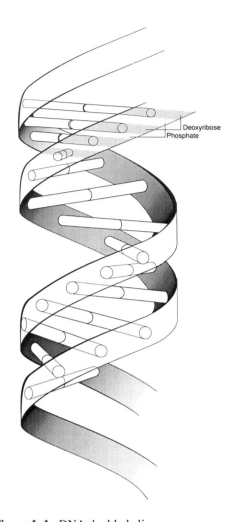

Figure 1–1. DNA double helix.

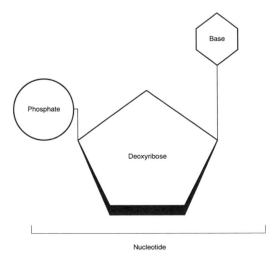

Figure 1–2. Structure of a nucleotide.

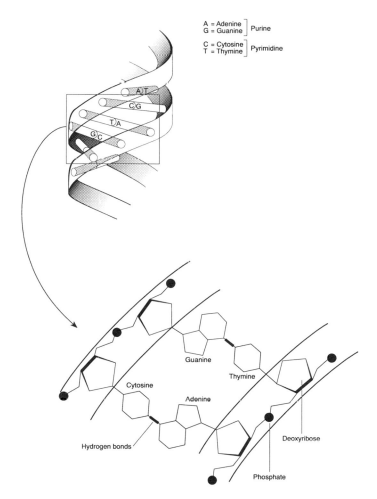

Figure 1–3. Stucture of a DNA molecule.

The genes themselves vary in size. The smallest known gene may be the alpha-globin gene, which is less than a thousand base pairs long.[7] This gene is responsible for producing a protein chain which combines with others to become hemoglobin, the oxygen-carrying molecule in red blood cells.[8] The largest known gene is the gene for dystrophin, which when defective can cause Duchenne muscular dystrophy, a genetic disease associated with progressive muscle weakness in boys that usually results in death by age 20.[9] The dystrophin gene is longer than 2 million base pairs.[10]

Humans have two corresponding versions, or two *alleles*, of most genes. Nearly every long thread of human DNA, containing several genes and other sequences, matches another thread with corresponding alleles. Each long thread is wound and folded around several proteins, like a sewing thread on a series of spools, until the DNA is coiled so tightly that it is condensed up to nearly 5,000–fold. The resulting complexes of DNA and proteins are called *chromosomes*.[11]

Every human being has 46 chromosomes, 44 of which occur in matched pairs, containing corresponding alleles. These 22 pairs are called *autosomes*, meaning any chromosome other than the sex chromosomes, which are labeled X and Y chromosomes. The X and Y chromosomes determine a person's gender. A female has two X chromosomes. A male has one X and one Y chromosome.[12]

Gene Function

Gene Expression

Each gene directs the cell in which it resides to produce a single protein or other product through a series of intracellular steps collectively called *gene expression*. Think of a gene as something like a written phrase of music and of each base as a single musical note. A specific series of notes prescribe a specific tune. Likewise, a specific series of bases *encode* a specific protein. Cells create proteins by expressing genes, much as musicians create music by playing the notes of the musical score.

The process of gene expression includes two major steps, *transcription* and *translation*. Through these steps, cells use genetic information to produce products, mainly proteins, that constitute cell structure and perform cell functions. The sequence of bases in each gene prescribes a specific sequence of amino acids, which are the building blocks of a protein.

Transcription

Transcription, the first step in gene expression, is a process in which a single-stranded molecule is created, with a base sequence complementary to the base sequence of the gene that is being expressed. The transcribed molecule is composed of ribonucleic acid (RNA), a compound which has the same bases as DNA, except that uracil (U) is substituted for thymine (T). U, like T, is a pyrimidine that specifically pairs with adenine (A).

Transcription occurs when the DNA double helix partially and transiently unwinds (the two strands disassociate), and an enzyme called *RNA polymerase II* recognizes a particular sequence of bases, called a *promoter*, that is present at the beginning of a gene on one or the other strand of DNA. Remember that the strand that contains the gene in question (the "sense" strand) is opposed by another strand of complementary DNA (called the "nonsense" strand). RNA polymerase II, which recognizes the promoter on the sense strand, uses the nonsense strand as a template. RNA polymerase II travels along the DNA in a linear fashion, lining up and connecting RNA nucleotides that complement the sequence of DNA nucleotides on the nonsense strand. The resulting single strand of RNA has a base sequence that is complementary to the base sequence of the nonsense DNA strand and matches the base sequence of the DNA sense strand[13] (Figure 1-4).

RNA has many roles in a cell, perhaps the most important of which is its role as a conveyor of the genetic information held in its sequence of bases, from the genes in the nucleus to the ribosomes, where protein synthesis occurs. Based upon its function, the species of RNA that performs this role is called *messenger RNA (mRNA)*.

Before the mRNA leaves the nucleus, it undergoes specific modifications that prepare it for its role in translation. These modifications, known as *mRNA processing*, include the addition of a *cap* and a *poly A tail* that mark the beginning and the end, respectively, of the mRNA. Small molecules, called *methyl groups* (consisting of a carbon and three hydrogen atoms), are attached to the mRNA,

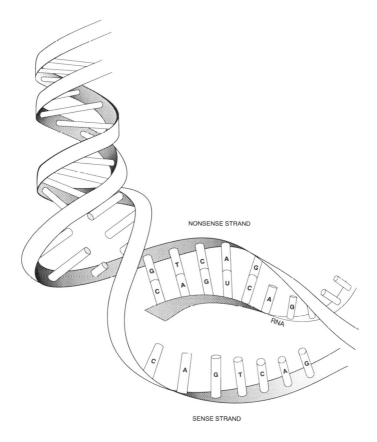

Figure 1–4. The RNA base sequence is complementary to the base sequence of the DNA nonsense strand.

possibly for the purpose of making them more stable and long-lived. Perhaps the most significant post-transcriptional modifications are those in which stretches of RNA are edited out of the transcript and the remaining pieces are spliced together. These sequences of DNA that are transcribed but excised before the transcript leaves the nucleus are called *introns*. Introns are apparently not necessary for translation. The portions of DNA corresponding to the mRNA sequences that are actually translated are called *exons*.[14]

Translation

After it is processed, the mRNA travels out of the nucleus to the ribosomes, where protein synthesis occurs. Every protein consists of one or more polypeptides (chains of amino acids) linked together in specific sequences. The sequence of amino acids in a polypeptide chain is determined by the sequence of bases in an mRNA. On the surface of each ribosome, mRNA is translated from the language of the genetic code into an amino acid sequence that constitutes a protein.

The genetic code has been entirely deciphered and charted by careful research (Table 1-1). Every possible sequence of three consecutive RNA bases, called a *triplet* or a *codon*, specifies a particular amino acid or a signal to stop translation. There are 64 possible codons, but only 20 amino acids, making for some overlap, or *degeneracy*, in the code; that is, several codons prescribe the same amino acids.[15]

Table 1–1. The Genetic Code

First Position (5' end)	Second Position				Third Position (3' end)
	U	*C*	*A*	*G*	
	PHE	SER	TYR	CYS	U
U	PHE	SER	TYR	CYS	C
	LEU	SER	Stop	Stop	A
	LEU	SER	Stop	TRP	G
	LEU	PRO	HIS	ARG	U
C	LEU	PRO	HIS	ARG	C
	LEU	PRO	GLN	ARG	A
	LEU	PRO	GLN	ARG	G
	ILE	THR	ASN	SER	U
A	ILE	THR	ASN	SER	C
	ILE	THR	LYS	ARG	A
	MET	THR	LYS	ARG	G
	VAL	ALA	ASP	GLY	U
G	VAL	ALA	ASP	GLY	C
	VAL	ALA	GLU	GLY	A
	VAL	ALA	GLU	GLY	G

Ribosomes are tiny protein factories, themselves composed of several types of proteins and RNAs. Ribosomes attach successively to an mRNA strand and catalyze the synthesis of polypeptide chains (Figure 1-5). Each ribosome translates the mRNA into protein by moving along the mRNA one codon at a time and facilitating the placement of a corresponding amino acid.[16]

Amino acids are actually carried to the polypeptide chains that are growing on the surface of ribosomes by special intermediary molecules called *transfer RNAs* (*tRNAs*). Every amino acid affiliates with a tRNA possessing a specific triplet base sequence (an *anticodon*) that is complementary to a particular mRNA codon. The tRNA anticodon and the mRNA codon pair up, assuring that the correct amino acid will be placed in sequence on a growing chain. When the ribosome reaches a stop codon, no tRNA presents itself; the ribosome releases the polypeptide chain and is itself released from the mRNA, ending translation.[17] The polypeptide chain eventually folds up and sometimes complexes with additional chains or other molecules, so the final protein is not a linear chain, but a tertiary structure.

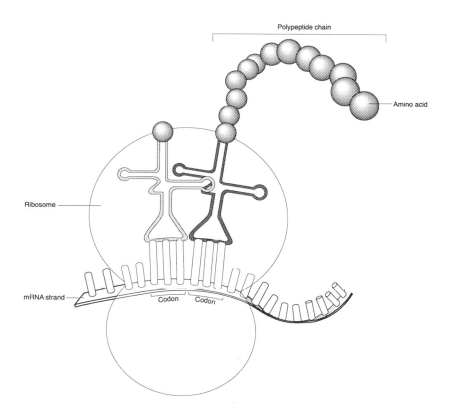

Figure 1–5. Translation of a protein.

Regulation of gene expression

Genes are expressed, and proteins thereby produced, in precise amounts and at particular times. In other words, gene expression is controlled, or *regulated*. As one noted textbook describes the regulation of gene expression, "[F]or harmonious and economic function of the cellular ensemble of enzymes it is absolutely essential that each gene produce neither more nor less than the amount of its product that promotes optimal growth."[18] Just as a musical score contains "tempo and expression marks" that direct the speed, loudness, and emotion of a piece of music, so DNA contains mechanisms for directing the timing and volume of protein production.

Gene expression may be regulated at any of several levels. Often, the initiation of transcription is the subject of regulation. *Repressor* proteins may attach to specific sequences of DNA and prevent the initiation of transcription, or *activators* may be required to start transcription. Then, the presence or absence of functioning repressors or activators determines whether transcription begins. The sequences of DNA with which regulatory proteins, such as repressors and activators, interact are called *regulatory sequences*.

There are many other mechanisms by which gene expression is regulated. Structural changes in the DNA may have an effect on gene expression by influencing the efficiency of gene transcription. Gene expression may be regulated by factors that limit or extend the stability and longevity of the transcript. Factors that affect the processing of RNA, the transport of mRNA to the ribosomes, the rate of translation, or even the processing and stability of the proteins themselves, can all be considered regulators of gene expression.[19]

The Role of Genes in Heredity

All of the cells in every person's body, except the sperm and egg cells, also called *gametes* or *germ cells*, contain a complete set of that person's genes, located on 46 chromosomes. Gametes are formed when diploid cells (containing 46 chromosomes) undergo a specific type of cell division called *meiosis*. (See Appendix A for a description of mitosis and meiosis.) During meiosis, pairs of chromosomes are divided so that the resulting germ cells (*haploid cells*) each have only 23 chromosomes (*diploid cells* have 46). Every germ cell contains half of each pair of the parent's autosomes plus either an X or a Y. Consequently, every germ cell contains one allele of each autosomal gene.

A germ cell does not, however, have merely one or another set of chromosomes that are identical to the chromosomes of the cell from which it is descended (its *precursor*). Rather, every germ cell receives a mixture of the genes that can be found on its precursor's pairs of chromosomes. This mixture is achieved when, before meiotic division occurs, a diploid cell's chromosomes line up next to each other and trade genes. The significance of this trading, or *crossing over*, is that parental genes sort somewhat independently. In other words, the integrity of parental chromosomes is not preserved, and each gamete has a novel set of 23 unique chromosomes rather than a novel set of 23 chromosomes which are individually identical to those contained in the diploid cells of the parent. (See Appendix A.)

During fertilization, two germ cells join to form a fertilized egg, or *zygote*, which has 46 chromosomes and two alleles of most genes (the exception being in boys who receive only one version of certain genes that are located on the X and Y chromosomes). Half of the zygote's genes are contributed by the mother's egg and half are contributed by the father's sperm. A zygote becomes a fetus and then a child through a series of cell divisions, during which its complete, unique genome is distributed to all of its descendant cells. The germ cells are thus the purveyors of heredity, passing genes from parents to child.

Based on this remarkable system, no child has a set of genes that is identical to either of his parents, but every child has a mixture of genes that includes one of two alleles from each parent. The information contained in these genes (also known as the *genotype*) encodes proteins that are responsible for the function of every cell in a person's body, and ultimately for that person's observable physical traits (known as his or her *phenotype*).

Genetic Disease

Sickle cell anemia is a disease phenotype that sheds light on both gene function and a gene's role in heredity. A genetic disease that occurs primarily in African blacks and their descendants, sickle cell anemia is caused by a single base change in the genes of its sufferers. The substitution of T for A alters the codon for a single amino acid in one of the polypeptide chains of an important red blood cell protein called *hemoglobin*. The codon change results in a substitution of one amino acid, valine, for another, glutamic acid, at the sixth position of the beta chain of hemoglobin (*beta globin*). This amino acid substitution affects a critical region of the hemoglobin protein so that it collapses when oxygen levels in the blood decrease, causing normally smooth, round red blood cells to crumple into the characteristic shape of a sickle. The sickled red blood cells impair blood circulation and cause obstructions, pain, and tissue damage.[20]

Remember that every person has two alleles of most genes, including the gene that encodes beta globin. When both alleles of a person's beta globin gene contain the critical base substitution, that person is considered *homozygous* for sickle cell anemia. A homozygote for sickle cell anemia exhibits the sickle cell anemia phenotype, that is, suffers from the disease. When only one of a person's two beta globin alleles contains the critical base substitution, that person is *heterozygous* for sickle cell anemia. A heterozygote's blood may contain some sickled cells, but he or she appears clinically normal. The single properly functioning beta globin gene encodes enough functional beta globin to prevent the person from suffering disease symptoms.[21]

Sickle cell anemia, one of many examples of diseases caused by a defect in a single gene, is known as a *recessive* disease. Recessive diseases occur only in individuals who are homozygous for the altered gene that causes a particular disease. Sufferers of recessive diseases have inherited two copies of a disease-causing gene, one from each parent. Most often, the parents are heterozygotes who do not suffer from any noticeable symptoms because they each have only one copy of the faulty gene.[22]

Recessive diseases belong to the genetic disease category known as *Mendelian* disease, named for the Austrian monk Gregor Mendel, who, in the 1860s, characterized the inheritance patterns of individual traits in the course of his work with pea plants. Mendelian diseases are those which result from a defect in a single gene (though it may be in both alleles in many cells), which have a large effect on a person's phenotype, and which are inherited in simple patterns (further described in Appendix B).[23]

Another category of Mendelian disease is *dominant* genetic disease. Dominant diseases are phenotypically manifested even when only one copy of the disease-causing allele is present and the other allele is functioning properly (that is, even when a person is heterozygous for that gene). An example of a dominant genetic disease is Huntington disease, which is characterized by personality changes and involuntary movements of the arms and legs.[24]

Besides Mendelian disease, three additional categories of genetic disease can be identified according to the role of their genetic components.[25] *Chromosomal disorders* involve the addition, deletion, or rearrangement of entire chromosomes or portions of chromosomes. These diseases necessarily concern numerous genes, because every chromosome contains many thousands of genes. Down syndrome, one well-known example of a chromosomal disorder, is caused by the presence of an extra chromosome 21.[26]

Multifactorial diseases involve multiple components, both environmental and genetic. Diabetes and hypertension, which both involve the interaction of genetic factors with environmental influences, are two examples of multifactorial diseases.[27]

The fourth category of genetic disease is *somatic cell genetic disease*. Unlike Mendelian diseases, chromosomal disorders, and multifactorial diseases, somatic cell diseases are not transmitted to subsequent generations through the *germ line* (via the germ cells). Diseases in this last category are caused by alterations of genes in specific somatic cells (cells other than those destined to become germ cells).[28] Examples of somatic cell genetic diseases include various cancers, some congenital malformations, and possibly autoimmune diseases.[29]

All of these types of genetic diseases have in common their origin from alterations, or *mutations*, in critical portions of important genes. Mutations that cause genetic diseases may arise spontaneously or as a result of environmental influences. They can be divided into several categories, based upon the alteration of DNA that they represent:[30] (1) *deletion mutations* involve the omission of relatively long stretches of DNA; (2) *insertion mutations* involve the addition of similar multibase sequences of DNA; (3) *point mutations* involve the substitution of one nucleotide for another (like the single base substitution that causes sickle cell anemia); and (4) *frameshift mutations* involve the addition or deletion of one or two nucleotides, which forces a regrouping of the three-base codons that are translated into amino acids (that is, a shift in the *reading frame*) and thereby completely changes the set of amino acids that are incorporated into a polypeptide chain during translation. Not every mutation causes disease. Many mutations occur in sequences of DNA that are not significant to the structure or function of vital gene products.

Although individual genetic diseases are often quite rare, collectively they are responsible for much human suffering. The 11th edition of Victor McKusick's well-known catalog of genetic disorders, *Mendelian Inheritance In Man*, published in 1994, lists 6,678 Mendelian traits and disorders.[31] Chromosomal, multifactorial, and somatic cell genetic disorders together are responsible for several times that number of human diseases. The desire to find effective and permanent cures for these genetic diseases has driven much of the gene therapy research that will be presented in the subsequent chapters.

Notes

1. United States, Congress, Office of Technology Assessment (OTA), *Human Gene Therapy: Background Paper* (Washington, DC: OTA, December 1984), p. 86.

2. Robert C. King and William D. Stansfield, *A Dictionary of Genetics* (4th ed.; New York: Oxford University Press, 1990), p. 216; Gunther S. Stent and Richard Calendar, *Molecular Genetics: An Introductory Narrative* (2nd ed.; San Francisco: W. H. Freeman and Company, 1978), p. 8.

3. In using words like "error," "malfunction," and "mutation," we have made a difficult choice. These words are all used to represent changes in DNA that can cause a gene to function in a way that is different from its function in most people and which can lead to untoward effects. They simplify that explanation, but also may carry immaterial connotations. Any implication that such DNA changes are categorically "bad" is unintended and hopefully refuted by the substance of this book.

We have encountered a similar problem with the word "normal." Any implication that normal DNA sequences are categorically "good" is not intended. The scientific term for a normally functioning gene is *wild type*, which also delivers extraneous messages that interfere with the term's basic significance.

4. James D. Watson, John Tooze, and David T. Kurtz, *Recombinant DNA: A Short Course* (New York: Scientific American Books, 1983), pp. 11–12.

5. Victor A. McKusick, *Mendelian Inheritance in Man: A Catalog of Human Genes and Genetic Disorders* (11th ed.; 2 vols.; Baltimore: Johns Hopkins University Press, 1994), p. xlv.

6. Ibid.

7. Ibid.

8. Eve K. Nichols, *Human Gene Therapy* (Cambridge, MA: Harvard University Press, 1988), p. 228.

9. Ibid., p. 224.

10. McKusick, op. cit., p. xlvi.

11. Thomas D. Gelehrter and Francis S. Collins, *Principles of Medical Genetics* (Baltimore: Williams & Wilkins, 1990), pp. 18–19.

12. Ibid.

13. Ibid., p. 14.

14. OTA, op. cit., pp. 48–49; Maxine Singer and Paul Berg, *Genes and Genomes: A Changing Perspective* (Mill Valley, CA: University Science Books, 1991), pp. 224–225.

15. Gelehrter and Collins, op. cit., pp. 15–17.

16. Singer and Berg, op. cit., pp. 33–34; Gelehrter and Collins, pp. 15–17.

17. Singer and Berg, op. cit., pp. 33–34; Gelehrter and Collins, pp. 15–17.

18. Stent and Calendar, op. cit, p. 667.

19. Gelehrter and Collins, op. cit., p. 90; Singer and Berg, op. cit., p. 34.

20. David Suzuki and Peter Knudtson, *Genethics: The Clash Between the New Genetics and Human Values* (Cambridge, MA: Harvard University Press, 1989), pp. 168–174; Gelehrter and Collins, p. 6.

21. Gelehrter and Collins, pp. 38–39.

22. Ibid.

23. Ibid., pp. 27–28.

24. Ibid., p. 208.

25. McKusick, op. cit., p. xxv.

26. Singer and Berg, op. cit., pp. 16–17; Gelehrter and Collins, op. cit., pp. 3–4.

27. Gelehrter and Collins, pp. 3–4; McKusick, op. cit., p. xxv.

28. King and Stansfield, op. cit., p. 294.

29. McKusick, op. cit., p. xxv.

30. Singer and Berg, op. cit., pp. 400–407; Nichols, op. cit., pp. 26–31.

31. McKusick, op. cit, pp. xvi–xvii.

2

Somatic Cell
Gene Therapy

Scientific Issues

Gene Therapy for ADA Deficiency

On September 14, 1990, the first officially sanctioned human somatic-cell gene-therapy experiment began. A 4-year-old girl was the first of two children to receive a dose of her own cells in which a functioning counterpart of her malfunctioning gene had been previously inserted. As early as December of the same year, and continuing through the end of the first phase of the experiment in July 1991, newspaper headlines dramatically cheered news of the experiment's success.[1]

The subjects of this successful gene therapy experiment were children suffering from a rare genetic disease called *adenosine deaminase* (*ADA*) *deficiency*. ADA deficiency arises from the malfunction of a gene expressed in bone marrow *stem cells*, long-lived cells that differentiate into multiple types of blood cells, including infection-fighting T and B cells (varieties of white blood cells). The malfunctioning ADA genes in these cells fail to produce functional versions of adenosine deaminase, an enzyme that normally metabolizes a compound called *deoxyadenosine*. Absent ADA, toxic levels of deoxyadenosine accumulate. T cells suffer the most from this buildup. These important infection-fighting cells are devastated, leaving the patient prey to infections which healthy individuals could easily withstand. Ultimately, most patients suffering from this rare disease die from infection unless a matched bone marrow donor can be found.[2] Unfortunately, matched donors are available for only about 30% of patients.[3] ADA-deficiency patients usually die before they reach the age of 2.[4]

ADA deficiency was an appropriate initial candidate for gene therapy for several reasons. First, researchers had long been convinced that even a small level of ADA production would be sufficient to operate as a cure for an ADA-deficient patient. They therefore did not have to achieve high expression levels in order to test the therapy. Additionally, the ADA gene is subject to relatively simple regulation, which made the achievement of appropriate ADA gene expression less complex than for other genes. Most significant was the hope that T cells armed with properly functioning ADA genes might have a selective advantage in the human body, allowing them to persist and multiply while noncorrected, ADA-deficient T cells expired.[5] Indeed, research had shown that human T cells, to which the ADA gene was added, survived in the bloodstreams of laboratory mice for months, while the cells with defective ADA genes died rapidly. The mouse experiments were evidence that T cells containing an inserted, functioning ADA gene were likely to thrive in patients suffering from ADA deficiency.[6]

In addition, numerous other animal experiments, in mice and in monkeys, had demonstrated that T cells could be successfully grown in vitro (literally, "in glass," meaning in a test tube), genetically altered, and reintroduced into animals where they would function appropriately as immune cells.[7] Although researchers had initially hoped to insert the functioning ADA gene into bone marrow stem cells, where the gene could be expected to persist indefinitely, they were, until recently, unable to purify the stem cells in the laboratory. Nevertheless, the T-cell results in animals were good enough to warrant a human experiment of the therapy.[8]

A team of investigators, led by National Institutes of Health doctors W. French Anderson, R. Michael Blaese, Kenneth W. Culver, and Steven Rosenberg, designed the first human gene therapy experiments in accordance with these extensive, preliminary animal experiments. During the human gene therapy experiment, doctors obtained blood from each ADA-deficient patient. The research team isolated T cells from these blood samples in the laboratory and grew the T cells in vitro. Then they inserted properly functioning ADA genes into the T cell using a process known as *transduction* in which an engineered RNA virus called a *retrovirus* carried the genes into the T cells (both retroviruses and transduction will be described below). Finally, doctors reinfused into each patient her (both are female) own altered T cells. The patients each received approximately six doses of transduced cells during the several-month first phase of the experiment.[9]

In conjunction with the gene therapy, the patients received a drug called *polyethyleneglycol (PEG)-ADA*, a version of the ADA enzyme itself. PEG-ADA had previously proven somewhat effective, but not effective enough to allow patients to fully regain immune function. Although able to decrease extracellular levels of deoxyadenosine, PEG-ADA cannot gain entrance to the T cells. Hence, PEG-ADA treatment by itself left the patients' T cells disabled. The investigators hoped that gene therapy would correct the T cells themselves and decrease intracellular levels of deoxyadenosine.[10]

The first scientific report on this initial gene therapy study was published in *Science* in October 1995.[11] Both young patients continue to receive PEG-ADA, although the dose has been reduced by more than half.[12] In laboratory measures of immune system function, both patients have shown improvement since the initiation of gene therapy in late 1990 and early 1991. In fact, the T-cell count for the younger of the two patients rose from below normal (about 500) to the normal range (1,200–1,800), and her blood levels for the enzyme ADA rose to about 50% of the levels in heterozygotes who carry one normal and one nonfunctioning ADA gene. The researchers estimate that about half of the T cells in the circulation of this younger patient carry the ADA gene.[13] In contrast, the older patient has much lower levels of ADA, and only 0.1–1.0% of her circulating T cells carry the ADA gene.[14]

More important than the laboratory values of these two patients is the effect of gene therapy plus PEG-ADA on their daily lives. Here is the researchers' summary of their clinical progress.

The effects of this treatment on the clinical well-being of these patients is more difficult to quantitate. Patient 1 [the younger patient], who had been kept in relative isolation in her home for her first 4 years, was enrolled in public kindergarten after 1 year on the protocol and has missed no more school because of infectious disease than her classmates or siblings. She has grown normally in height and weight and is considered to be normal by her parents. Patient 2 was regularly attending public school while receiving PEG-ADA treatment alone and has continued to do well clinically. Chronic sinusitis and headaches, which had been a recurring problem for several years, cleared completely a few months after initiation of the protocol.[15]

The same issue of *Science* in which the U.S. ADA study was reported also included a report by Italian researchers on their study of gene therapy in two young children with ADA deficiency. The Italian research team was led by Claudio Bordignon of the Scientific Research Institute H. S. Raffaele in Milan. Both Italian patients had been started on enzyme therapy with PEG-ADA at the age of 2 years, and both had "failed"—that is, their immune systems were not adequately protecting them against infection—after treatment with PEG-ADA alone.[16] In the Italian study the two patients received both genetically modified T cells and genetically modified bone marrow cells plus ongoing support with PEG-ADA. Three years after the start of gene therapy in patient 1 (at age 5) and 2½ years after the start of treatment in patient 2 (at age 4), both patients are doing well clinically. The Italian researchers report that the genetically modified T cells have gradually died off after remaining in the children's circulation for 6–12 months but that the percentage of new T cells produced by genetically modified bone marrow progenitor cells is gradually increasing.[17]

The news media have greeted these two gene therapy studies with cautious optimism. For example, the headline of the story announcing the *Science* article on the U.S. study read, "Gene Therapy's First Success Is Claimed, But Doubts

Remain."[18] These doubts have to do mainly with two features of the studies performed to date. First, for understandable reasons the researchers have been reluctant to withdraw PEG-ADA from children who are doing well on a combination of PEG-ADA and (past) gene therapy. Second, the experimental step of removing, selecting, and expanding the number of T cells may have a beneficial effect for patients, in addition to the beneficial effects of the genetic modification itself. Further research will help to resolve these remaining questions.[19]

Important Features of the First U.S. Gene Therapy Study

The disease selected for the initial research. During the late 1970s and early 1980s considerable discussion was devoted to deciding which diseases would be the best targets for early gene therapy attempts. For example, in 1977 molecular biologist David Baltimore sketched a scenario for gene therapy using sickle cell anemia as his example.[20] However, in the 1980s diseases in which a single enzyme was missing in patients came to the fore, in part because the genes involved in the gene therapy would not need to be so precisely regulated as they would be in the treatment of a hemoglobin disorder like sickle cell anemia. In other words, new genes could be introduced into a patient's body and, even if the genes produced more of the missing enzyme than the patient's body needed, the patient would not be harmed. The excess enzyme would simply be eliminated from the patient's body like any other waste matter.

The target cells selected. Before the first gene therapy study was undertaken, there was considerable discussion of the target cells into which new genes could be introduced. The assumption was always that the cells would be removed from the patient's body, genetically modified in the laboratory, and then returned to the patient. Skin cells, or fibroblasts, were sometimes mentioned as possible targets for gene therapy. In a long preliminary proposal submitted for review in early 1987, W. French Anderson and his colleagues suggested that bone marrow cells might be the best targets.[21] However, the harvesting of bone marrow is a relatively invasive and painful procedure for the donor; it involves the introduction of a large needle into the hip bones, from which the marrow is removed. When Anderson, Blaese, Rosenberg, and Culver sat down to design their first actual gene therapy protocol, they decided that white blood cells, specifically the T cells, would be better targets. The harvesting of these cells would be less traumatic for the patient, and there was at least a hint in studies with mice that T cells that had the ADA gene survived longer than cells that lacked the gene.

As their research continued, the Blaese–Anderson group decided to aim their *vectors* (delivery vehicles) at another kind of cell that is closely related to the T cell. In fact, stem cells are the "parents" that give rise to several different types of blood cells, including T cells. The researchers reasoned that if they could introduce the ADA gene into even a few of these stem cells, all of the offspring of these parental cells would contain the previously missing gene. In the study with young children, Blaese and his colleagues attempted to perform stem cell therapy with one of the two female patients—without apparent success. The companion study in newborns modified only stem cells derived from the umbilical cords of the infants.

It is important to note that all of the proposed target cells for the earliest studies of gene therapy have been somatic, or nonreproductive, cells. The new genes introduced into those cells are not likely to escape and "spread" to the sperm or egg cells of the recipient. Thus, the new genes will probably not be passed on to the descendants of the patient who receives this experimental treatment.

The vector employed. The ADA gene therapy experiment involved the addition of genes to cells which had been removed from a patient's body and grown in vitro. The genes were delivered to the cells in vitro by a clever manipulation of the naturally occurring RNA viruses called retroviruses. Retroviruses are so named because upon entering cells, they use an enzyme called *reverse transcriptase* to transcribe their genomes from RNA to DNA, a kind of "backward" transcription.[22] These resourceful viruses have the ability to integrate into the host genome, thereby tricking the host cell into treating them as if they were part of the host cell's own DNA.

Retroviruses can be virulent, multiplying and destroying their host cells. In fact human immunodeficiency virus (HIV), the virus responsible for acquired immune deficiency syndrome (AIDS), is one example of a deadly retrovirus. However, retroviruses can be engineered so that their harmful sequences are deleted and the sequences that allow them to integrate into a host genome are preserved. By replacing the deleted sequences with genes that a researcher wants to deliver to cells, he or she can exploit the retrovirus's ability to efficiently enter cells and deliver genes to host chromosomes. There is a sort of poetic justice in using these viruses that are themselves so manipulative of their hosts' machinery.

Retroviruses are comprised of RNA and protein. The fully assembled retroviral package (for any virus, called a *virion*) contains two identical strands of RNA, structural proteins, and reverse transcriptase. All of these core components are surrounded by an envelope, or *coat*, consisting of *glycoprotein* (a protein that contains small amounts of carbohydrate[23]), which is responsible for attaching to and allowing the virus to penetrate cells.

The retroviral genome (that is, one complete set of genetic information contained in the retroviral RNA) consists of three genes and a regulatory sequence.[24] The three genes are *gag, pol,* and *env*. Gag encodes several structural proteins derived from an initially expressed product that is cleaved after translation. Pol encodes reverse transcriptase as well as other enzymes. Env encodes the envelope glycoprotein. The regulatory sequence, which is called a *long terminal repeat (LTR)*, contains sequences vital for regulation of RNA synthesis, transcript processing, and integration of the virus into the host genome.[25] In addition, the genome contains a nucleotide sequence called *psi* that must be present on a strand of RNA in order for that strand to be packaged as a virus (Figure 2-1).

Its normal life cycle makes the retrovirus a good medium for delivering genes into cells. The virion binds to membrane receptors on a host cell and the retrovirus enters the cell, leaving behind its glycoprotein envelope. Once inside the cell, the retrovirus uses reverse transcriptase to transcribe a single-stranded *complementary DNA (cDNA)* molecule from its own single strand of RNA. The host cell's enzymes cannot discriminate the viral cDNA from host DNA, and they synthesize from the cDNA template a double-stranded DNA molecule with an LTR at each end. This DNA molecule integrates into the host genome, becoming what is called a *provirus*. The provirus is transmitted along with the rest of the host genome to daughter cells when the host divides. At another stage in its life cycle, the retrovirus may be reproduced and repackaged separately from the host genome, thereby reasserting its virulence[26] (Figure 2-2).

Molecular biologists use recombinant DNA techniques to obtain the proviral DNA form of the retroviral genome and to replace gag, pol, and env with the nonviral gene they desire to use for gene therapy. They preserve the LTR sequences which are necessary for integration, but without gag, pol, and env, the retrovirus cannot package itself into a virion after transcription. With psi remaining, however, these *recombinant* retroviruses *can* be packaged by researchers, who transcribe RNA genomes from the altered proviral DNA and supply an independent source of gag, pol, and env gene products[27] (Figure 2-3).

After disabling and packaging retroviruses for use as *vectors*, researchers use them to transduce cells in vitro, that is, to deliver the inserted gene to recipient cells, where the vector integrates but is unable to reproduce itself. The integrated provirus is passed along to daughter cells when the cell divides, resulting in a whole colony of cells that contain the added gene.[28] In the ADA gene therapy experiment, this process was used to insert ADA genes into T cells or stem cells, which were then infused into the patients.

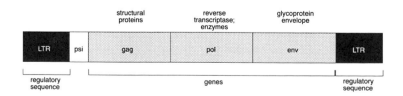

Figure 2–1. Retroviral genome.

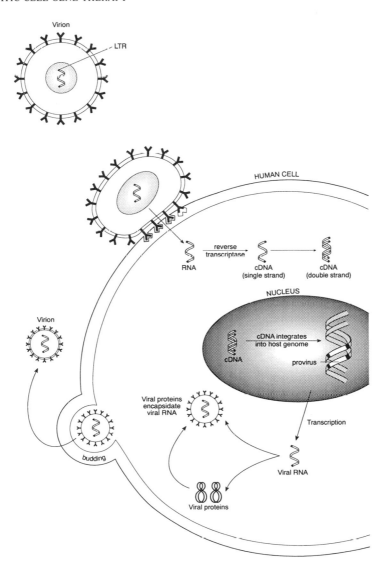

Figure 2–2. Life cycle of a retrovirus.

Gene addition as the basic strategy. The gene therapy study that seeks to treat patients with severe combined immune deficiency (SCID) adds a functioning copy of the ADA gene to as many T cells or stems cells as possible. With current techniques it is possible to achieve only random integration of the vector and the new gene into the genome of each cell. Thus, except for the offspring of stem cells and the daughter cells of T cells, every integration site is likely to be unique. In the future, researchers hope to be able to achieve genuine gene replacement or gene repair (see Appendix E), but at present gene addition is the most that can be accomplished.

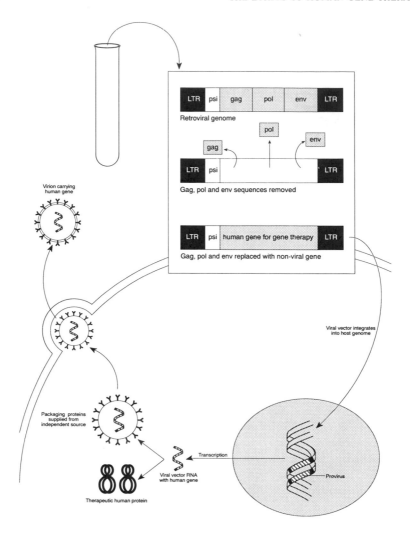

Figure 2–3. Recombinant retrovirus that can be used for gene therapy.

The involvement of industry. The retroviral vector used in the initial gene therapy study had been developed by a company called Genetic Therapy, Incorporated (GTI). However, all of the clinical research in the study has been conducted either at the NIH Clinical Center or at hospitals in California. In 1990, when the study was initiated, the four primary researchers, W. French Anderson, R. Michael Blaese, Kenneth Culver, and Steven A. Rosenberg, held full-time appointments at the National Institutes of Health (NIH). Blaese and Rosenberg remain at NIH, while Anderson and Culver have moved to a faculty position at the University of Southern California and a research position with OncorPharm, respectively. The initial study has been funded primarily by NIH; GTI has made a substantial investment in developing and certifying the vector.[29]

Developments in Gene Therapy since 1990

Five years after the treatment of the first gene therapy patient in an approved pro-tocol there are 100 protocols that have either been approved by the NIH Recom-binant DNA Advisory Committee or that are under review at the U.S. Food and Drug Administration. The target diseases in these 100 studies are the following (numbers refer to number of studies):

Cancers of various types: 63 (63%)
HIV infection/AIDS: 12 (12%)
Genetic diseases: 22 (22%)
Other diseases: 3 (3%)
    Rheumatoid arthritis: 1
    Peripheral artery disease: 1
    Arterial restenosis: 1

The category "Genetic Diseases" can be further subdivided among the following disorders (numbers refer to number of studies):

Cystic fibrosis: 12
Gaucher disease (type I): 3
SCID due to adenosine deaminase (ADA) deficiency: 1
Familial hypercholesterolemia: 1
Alpha 1-antitrypsin deficiency: 1
Fanconi anemia: 1
Hunter syndrome (mild form): 1
Chronic granulomatous disease: 1
Purine nucleoside phosphorylase (PNP) deficiency: 1

Generalizations about the Later Gene Therapy Studies

Target cells. As we have noted, Blaese, Anderson, and associates had sought initially to add the gene for adenosine deaminase (ADA) to the type of white blood cell called the T cell. Later they added the gene to stem cells derived from the circulatory system of one of their female patients and from the umbilical cords of their three newborn patients. Other researchers took aim at a wide variety of *somatic*, or *nonreproductive*, cells. Many of the cystic fibrosis protocols tried to modify the cells on the surface of the lungs. Other protocols have targeted liver cells, tumor-infiltrating white blood cells, blood vessel cells, and cancer cells. Approximately two-thirds of the first 100 gene therapy studies treated the cell's outside the recipient patient's body and then introduced the genetically modified cells into the patient through one of several means. In these studies the cells were said to have been treated *ex vivo*. In the remaining one-third of the protocols, the vector and gene were joined outside the patient's body but only were united with the patient's cells inside the patient's body. For example, in the cystic fibrosis studies, the vector–gene combination is sometimes introduced into the lungs through an aerosol spray. These cells are treated in vivo.

Vectors. As one might expect, different target cells sometimes require different kinds of vectors. The first changes from the traditional retroviral vectors came with the early cystic fibrosis protocols. For these studies researchers initially chose a virus that causes flu-like respiratory infections, the *adenovirus*. Again the virus was domesticated to reduce the likelihood that it would make the recipient ill or spread infection to the people around the recipient. Other studies have used the adeno-associated virus, or AAV. Some researchers have forsworn viral vectors and used other methods to place new genes into target cells. One of the most-used methods encapsulates the new DNA in fatty spheres called *liposomes* and uses injections to move these spheres close to the target cells. (For detailed information on additional methods for delivering genes to cells, see Appendix C.)

Researchers are generally agreed that there is currently no one ideal vector for all situations. Each of the available vectors has some advantages and some disadvantages. New vectors are on the drawing board in many laboratories. One researcher, Francis Collins, has even proposed the construction of a human artificial chromosome as a vector for the future.[30] Presumably such a synthetic chromosome would take its place beside the 46 already in the patient's cells and would include all of the control mechanisms that are present in the original 46.

Gene addition. In gene therapy protocols 2–100, gene addition continues to be the only approach. Gene replacement or gene repair methods are not sufficiently advanced to be proposed for human studies.

Industry involvement. Between 1990 and 1995 private industry became increasingly involved in gene therapy at two levels. As in the original ADA study, commercial firms have continued to develop vectors and to supply them to researchers. About two-thirds of the first 100 studies received their vectors from companies; the remaining one-third secured vectors from academic institutions. In addition, several companies have become industrial sponsors of human gene therapy trials, especially the studies involving larger numbers of patients. Among these companies are Genetic Therapy Inc., Genzyme, Viagene, and Vical.

One other mode of industry participation in gene therapy deserves at least brief mention. In March of 1995 NIH was granted a broad patent on ex vivo gene therapy—that is, on gene therapy that modifies human cells outside the patient's body.[31] NIH had agreed in advance that this patent, when issued, would be licensed exclusively to Genetic Therapy, Inc. (GTI). Any other researcher or company that wishes to use the ex vivo method of modifying cells to develop a commercial product will need to purchase a sublicense from GTI. How this patent will affect the future of gene therapy remains to be seen.

Detailed Information about the Later Studies

Familial hypercholesterolemia: in vitro. *Familial hypercholesterolemia (FH)* is a genetic disease associated with astronomically high cholesterol levels in its sufferers. Patients who have the most severe form of FH can have cholesterol concentrations four or five times as high as healthy individuals. Most FH patients die prematurely from heart attacks.[32]

The abnormally high levels of cholesterol in FH patients arc thc result of malfunctioning genes responsible for directing the production of cellular receptors that capture and remove low-density lipoprotein (LDL) cholesterol from the bloodstream. Without the help of the LDL receptors normally present on the surface of liver cells, FH patients are unable to clear LDL cholesterol from their bloodstreams.

James M. Wilson, chief of Molecular Medicine and Genetics at the University of Pennsylvania, first worked with ADA-deficiency and Lesch-Nyhan syndrome patients but became interested in pursuing gene therapy for FH after reading about a well-known FH patient named Stormy Jones who was near death before being cured by a combined liver–heart transplant. Wilson realized that if he could devise a way to introduce the LDL receptor gene into the liver cells of FH patients without a full-scale liver transplant, he could increase the number of FH patients able to receive treatment (matched livers are not available for every FH patient) and reduce the invasiveness of treatment (liver transplants require immunosuppression while gene therapy does not).[33]

Wilson's gene therapy experiment was successfully tested first in *Watanabe rabbits*, animals which suffer from the equivalent of human FH. The human experiment began in June 1992. It involved several steps. The patients were placed under anesthesia before surgery. Fifteen to fifty percent of the patients' livers were removed and a catheter was placed into the portal vein, which supplies the liver with blood. In the laboratory, liver cells called *hepatocytes* were isolated and cultured in vitro. Forty eight hours later, these cells were exposed to retroviral vectors containing properly functioning LDL receptor genes. The exposure lasted 12–18 hours, after which the cells were washed, harvested, and reinfused into each patient's liver via the catheter previously inserted. Finally, the catheter was removed.[34]

Eighteen months after treatment of a 28-year-old woman, the first patient under the FH gene therapy protocol, Wilson and his colleagues reported that the patient had significantly reduced LDL levels and that the study had demonstrated "the feasibility, safety and potential efficacy of *ex vivo* liver directed gene therapy in humans." At the time of their published report, however, it was still unclear whether the patient's improved LDL levels would result in an improved clinical outcome. The researchers were satisfied at least that the patient's coronary artery disease had not progressed during the 18 months since the gene therapy procedure was performed. In addition, they announced that this FH gene therapy represented the first example of a stable gene-therapy-derived correction of a "therapeutic endpoint," in contrast to the ADA gene therapy trials, which required repeated administration of genetically modified cells.[35]

Like Anderson's ADA-deficiency gene therapy, Wilson's FH experiment involves in vitro gene transfer and requires that patients' cells be removed from their bodies before the functioning genes are administered. Wilson believes that gene therapy will not achieve real medical relevance until genes can be bottled, distributed, and then administered in vivo by ordinary medical practitioners. In accordance with this vision, Wilson spends most of his time working on the development of what he calls *injectable genes*.[36]

Still working with FH and genes expressed in the liver, Wilson and his colleague George Y. Wu, of the University of Connecticut, have developed an artificial DNA virus. Their constructed virus consists of DNA, including a functional LDL receptor gene, coated with protein that is recognizable by liver cells. Within minutes after this complex is infused into the ear vein of Watanabe rabbits, liver cells scoop up the protein from circulation and pick up the DNA along with it. The Watanabe rabbits' cholesterol levels fall, but only transiently because the injected gene is soon degraded. Wilson and his colleagues are pursuing a strategy for accomplishing prolonged or permanent LDL receptor gene activity by following the gene injection with stimulation of liver cell growth. When genes are taken up by cells during cell division, the genes are more likely to integrate into the host genome and result in stable expression.[37]

Wilson's injectable genes are not yet ready for human trials because of a number of limitations, including the risk that some of the injected genes may be randomly picked up by cells other than liver cells, possibly resulting in LDL expression in inappropriate cells. Nevertheless, when perfected, in vivo gene therapy will have several advantages over gene therapy mediated by gene transfer into cells in vitro. It will allow the delivery of genes to appropriate cells without invasive procedures, and will reach a greater number of cells than those which can be removed, thereby holding out the promise of more complete amelioration of disease symptoms.[38]

Hereditary emphysema. Hereditary emphysema is a lung disease caused by a mutation in the gene that encodes an enzyme called alpha 1–antitrypsin (AAT). Normally, AAT protects the lungs from damage by neutrophil elastase, a powerful enzyme which is capable of destroying lung tissue. Without functioning AAT, a person's lungs are easy prey for neutrophil elastase. Current treatments for this disease, which causes progressive respiratory impairment and a shortened life-span, are effective but extremely expensive.

Ronald G. Crystal of New York Hospital-Cornell Medical Center and his collaborators have experimented with two different gene therapy alternatives that might be used to treat AAT deficiency.[39] Crystal's early AAT experiments involved inserting the AAT gene into mouse T cells and injecting the T cells into mice. Subsequent injections of substances designed to stimulate the immune system caused the T cells to proliferate. Crystal's group theorized that they would be able to induce the same proliferation of modified T cells in patients and, using aerosolized antigens, draw the AAT-expressing T cells to the patient's lungs, where AAT was required.[40]

In more recent experiments, Crystal's team aerosolized viral vectors carrying the AAT gene and sprayed them directly into the lungs of rats, where they transduced epithelial cells that lined the bronchial tubes. After 6 weeks, the AAT gene still persisted in the rats—promising evidence that the therapy could work in human AAT-deficiency patients. Crystal's team used recombinant adenoviruses. Adenoviruses were advantageous for many reasons, including the fact that they normally infect human respiratory cells and have a proven safety record as human vaccine viruses.[41]

Cystic fibrosis. Gene therapy holds promise for another common inherited lung disease, cystic fibrosis. Cystic fibrosis (CF) is one of the most common genetic diseases.[42] The gene responsible for CF, the cystic fibrosis transmembrane conductance regulator gene (CFTR), normally encodes a protein that helps transport ions (electric charge) across cell membranes. When this gene is defective, mucus-producing cells cannot access normal quantities of water. As a consequence, these cells produce thick, sticky mucus that chokes the lungs and other organs, harboring bacteria and leading to life-threatening infections.[43]

Delivering aerosolized genes directly to the lungs of CF patients may prove to be a nonintrusive and effective therapy.[44] Several research teams, including Crystal's, are working on experiments that use the adenovirus which naturally infects the tissue lining the lung (the *lung epithelium*) to deliver normal copies of the defective gene responsible for CF. Other groups have already succeeded in correcting the genetic defect in vitro in cells taken from CF patients.[45]

In addition, using adenoviral vectors, researchers have applied the normal CFTR gene to the nasal epithelia of CF patients, thereby correcting their defective ion channel without any serious inflammatory response and without replication of the adenovirus.[46]

Researchers would like to be able to use AAV as a vector for gene therapy in CF patients. AAV naturally infects the epithelial cells of the respiratory tract and the gastrointestinal tract. It can be produced in high concentrations in solution and it is nonpathogenic in its normal form. It also usually integrates into a specific, preferred chromosomal location, lowering the risk of insertional mutagenesis. Researchers have conducted animal trials and have submitted a protocol for a human trial to assess the usefulness of the AAV vector as a method for delivering the CFTR gene.

Additional delivery systems under scrutiny for CF gene therapy include retroviral vectors, liposomes (for a brief description of liposomes, see Appendix C), and receptor-mediated endocytosis (a method which involves attaching DNA to a molecule that binds to a specific cellular receptor, where it is internalized by the host cell).[47]

As of late 1995, 12 human CF gene therapy protocols have been submitted to regulatory bodies for approval, and 10 human trials are in progress or completed. Based on all of the current research, one reviewer has predicted that an effective gene therapy for CF will be available by 1999.[48]

Coronary artery disease. Sufferers of coronary artery disease, whether genetically derived or not, might be helped by the addition of genes encoding proteins that dissolve artery-clogging substances. A few different groups have developed techniques for adding such genes to the cells lining the inside of artery walls.

Judith L. Swain and colleagues at Duke University Medical Center have successfully inserted genes directly into the femoral arteries of the legs of several dogs, using a catheter to deliver the gene-fortified solution. For their experiment, they used luciferase genes, which encode an enzyme normally responsible for giving fireflies their glow. After a few days, the glow of the luciferase enzyme in surgically removed tissue allowed the researchers to easily detect that the added genes had not only entered the arterial cells, but also turned on and expressed.[49]

Elizabeth Nabel, Gregory Plautz, and Gary Nabel, of the University of Michigan Medical School, achieved similar results using a different gene in the arteries of pigs. They had success using both in vitro and in vivo techniques. In 1989, the Nabel team showed that endothelial cells could be genetically altered in vitro and then stably implanted on the arterial walls of Yucatan minipigs, where they expressed a recombinant gene.[50]

In September 1990, the Nabel group reported the results of an experiment in which they used a double-balloon catheter to deliver a viral vector containing a marker gene encoding a stainable protein directly into pig arteries. The two balloons blocked the artery on both sides of a small space into which the vector was flushed, thereby containing the vector in a protected space, where it transduced arterial endothelial cells. Even as long as 21 weeks later, the pigs' arterial cells still produced the stainable gene product.[51] The Nabel group achieved similar results using liposome transfection, demonstrating that, whether by transduction or transfection, they could deliver a recombinant gene to a specific site in vivo.[52]

Using methods for transducing or transfecting endothelial cells, researchers hope one day to be able to deliver to patients not just marker genes, but helpful genes that produce, for example, clot-preventing proteins. The same techniques could be used also for treatment of other illnesses in addition to artery disease. For instance, the addition of functioning genes to artery endothelial cells might be a workable, future mechanism for delivering clotting factors to the blood of hemophilia patients or for dispensing insulin to diabetics.[53]

Cancer. Cancer is a generic name for a "class of diseases characterized by uncontrolled cellular growth."[54] It is now the "leading cause of death for women in the United States and, if trends continue, will be the overall leading cause of death in the United States by the year 2000."[55] Scientists have identified several environmental and genetic causes of cancer, including tobacco (the primary cause). Because many of the causes of cancer are associated with lifestyle choices, prevention research contributes importantly to the fight against cancer.[56] Complementary research in cancer treatment has led to the development of a variety of different theories which involve the use of gene therapy as a cancer treatment. All of these include attempts to specifically target cancer cells for destruction or arrest. More than 50 clinical trials of gene therapy for the treatment of cancer are currently underway.

The first cancer gene therapy proposal actually became one of the first gene therapy experiments attempted in humans (shortly after the ADA experiment). The experiment, led by Dr. Steven A. Rosenberg, chief of surgery at the National Cancer Institute, involved an attempt to genetically engineer cancer patients' own cells to dispense products that destroyed their tumors.

Rosenberg removed naturally occurring white blood cells called tumor infiltrating lymphocytes (TILs) from patients suffering from malignant melanoma, a deadly skin cancer. These TILs have the ability to specifically home in on tumors growing in the patients' bodies. Using retroviral vectors in vitro, Rosenberg's team inserted into the TILs a gene that encoded tumor necrosis factor (TNF), a protein shown to vigorously fight tumors in mice. The TILs were then returned to the patients' bodies. It was hoped the engineered TILs would deliver the inserted TNF genes specifically to malignant tissue, where the genes would direct the production of TNF and destroy the patients' tumors. The human trial, which began on January 29, 1991, remained inconclusive in July 1991, when it was reported that Rosenberg and his colleagues had experienced difficulty in achieving persistent in vivo gene expression. Although Rosenberg said it was too early to tell whether the patients were benefiting from the gene therapy experiment, he did announce that none of the patients had been harmed.[57]

The second human-cancer gene therapy experiment involved genetic alteration of patients' cancer cells that was expected to induce cancer sufferers' own immune systems to mount an attack on their tumors. This line of human research was based in large part on the compelling work of Drew Pardoll, of Johns Hopkins University. Working in mice, Pardoll and his team inserted genes for an immune system chemical called *interleukin-4 (IL-4)* into kidney cancer cells that had been removed from the mice's own spontaneously arising tumors. They reintroduced the engineered tumor cells into the mice and found that in addition to rejecting and destroying the engineered tumor cells, the mice immune systems mounted attacks which destroyed the parent tumors.[58]

Rosenberg and his co-workers later tested this new gene therapy approach to cancer in humans, again working with melanoma patients. They removed tumor cells from the patients and, after growing them in laboratory cultures, inserted into them genes for TNF or interleukin-2. Interleukin-2, like TNF, is an immune system chemical that battles tumors. After readministering the engineered cells to the patients, the Rosenberg team anticipated that the tumor cells containing the added genes would stimulate an elevated immune system response in vivo before dying off.[59]

A similar human experiment, using liposomes to transfect tumor cells in vivo, was proposed in October 1991. A group led by Gary Nabel (University of Michigan) proposed to directly inject cancer patients' tumors with liposomes containing a gene that encodes HLA-B7, a protein that stimulates tissue rejection. The Nabel group hopes that tumor cells will take up and express the HLA-B7 gene, causing those cells to be recognized as foreign by the patients' immune systems.[60]

A third line of inquiry arises from basic research into the molecular genetics of cancer. During the 1980s and into the 1990s, accumulating evidence has suggested that the normal, controlled growth of cells is regulated by two contrary types of genes. One type, genes that promote the growth of cells, are called *proto-oncogenes*, or when they go awry, *oncogenes*. Certain mutations of proto-oncogenes activate them, turning them into oncogenes and fostering uncontrolled cell growth. Activated oncogenes are almost always dominant, switching on unregulated cell growth even when present in heterozygous form.[61]

Later research has unearthed counterposing genes, descriptively named *tumor suppressor genes*. Genetic mutations that inactivate tumor suppressor genes destroy the limitations they impose on cell growth and allow the unsuppressed growth of cancer cells. Such mutations may be inherited, but the great majority of them appear to be somatic.[62] Tumor-suppressor genes act recessively; both alleles must be knocked out by mutation before a cell becomes cancerous.[63] The multiplying discoveries of and about tumor-suppressor genes has generated research and speculation on the possibility of harnessing them for cancer gene therapy.[64]

Early research results have been promising. The *retinoblastoma (RB) gene* encodes a tumor suppressor protein that has been found inactivated in several types of cancer, including breast, lung, and prostate cancers. Robert Bookstein and his colleagues at the University of California at San Diego have shown that adding functioning RB genes to human prostate cancer cells suppresses the ability of those cells to participate in tumor formation when the cells are implanted in mice. Human prostate cancer cells without the added genes readily form tumors in the mice. Bookstein has postulated that at some future time, a therapy for cancer will evolve that is based on the addition of functioning RB genes or their RB protein products to cancer cells.[65]

Perhaps even more hopeful are the results obtained in experiments involving the tumor suppressor gene *p53*. Mutations in the p53 gene are the most frequently observed genetic alterations in human cancers.[66] Various p53 mutations have been found in colon cancers, breast cancers, lymphomas, leukemias, lung cancers, and esophageal cancers, among others.[67] Surprisingly, the p53 gene has the capacity to act as an oncogene as well as a failed repressor when it undergoes certain mutations. In other words, it sometimes actually switches from suppression to stimulation of cell division.[68] Researchers do not have a complete understanding of the p53 gene and its activities, but at least one interesting model has been suggested: While normal p53 works transiently in conjunction with a complex of other molecules, certain mutants of p53 may attach too tightly to the other molecules, sequestering them from their usual activities and leaving the cell without any of the active complexes that it needs for negative growth regulation.[69]

A team of researchers led by Bert Vogelstein, of The Johns Hopkins University School of Medicine, has demonstrated that the normal human p53 gene can specifically repress the growth of human colorectal cancer cells in vitro.[70] Another team, at Temple University, has found that the normal p53 gene can halt the growth of brain cancer cells in vitro.[71] It is hoped that continuing research will result in a mechanism for using functioning p53 genes to stop the growth of cancer cells in vivo in the many patients whose uncontrolled cell growth is a result of mutant p53. At least four human-cancer gene-therapy proposals aimed at modifying the expression of tumor-suppressor genes have been submitted to regulatory bodies; several have received approval as of this writing.

A group of researchers led by Edward H. Oldfield, a neurosurgeon at the National Institutes of Health has begun an experiment with people who have incurable, malignant brain tumors. The gene therapy strategy involves injecting the brain tumors with cells that have been genetically engineered to produce a vector containing a drug-sensitivity gene. It is hoped that this gene will be transferred into the tumor cells and make them sensitive to the drug ganciclovir (GCV). GCV is nontoxic to normal tissues, but will kill cells that express the gene in question.[72]

Other researchers have applied an inverse theory in designing human-cancer gene therapy trials. They have transferred drug resistance genes into human subjects' noncancerous cells for the purpose of protecting these normal cells from the effects of chemotherapy.[73]

Researchers are also testing in humans a gene therapy strategy called *antisense* gene therapy. The antisense strategy involves administering to cancer sufferers vectors that express RNA molecules which specifically block the function of certain genes that promote cancer growth. The antisense RNA molecules block gene expression by binding with the complementary base pairs of the targeted gene's transcript. Researchers hope that vectors expressing antisense RNA will be able to stop the growth and spread of cancers cells in patients.[74]

AIDS. AIDS is a somatic cell genetic disease that, in some respects, resembles ADA deficiency. AIDS is associated with a person's infection by HIV, which causes HIV-infected patients to suffer immune system impairment, resulting in increased infections and an increased risk of developing cancer. Several gene therapy strategies for treating HIV infection are being studied in animal models or have been proposed for human clinical trials.

One strategy that has already entered second-generation human clinical trials was originally proposed in 1993. This study involves administering retroviral vectors containing a gene coding for an HIV envelope protein to HIV-infected individuals. Scientists hope that the vector will trigger immune responses in HIV-infected patients. Specifically, it is hoped that their bodies will produce T cells which target and kill cells infected with viruses.[75]

Philip Greenberg, of the University of Washington, along with his research team, proposed in October 1991 to use gene therapy techniques to augment a bone marrow transplant treatment for HIV infection and one of its associated cancers, lymphoma. The treatment first entailed removing some of a patient's T cells—those cells with a specific ability to fight HIV infection. The harvested T cells were transduced in vitro with a gene (the HyTK gene) that caused those T cells to self-destruct if the patient were later exposed to particular drugs. Then doctors irradiated the patient's bone marrow in order to destroy both the patient's lymphoma and HIV-infected cells. Next, the patient received a bone marrow transplant from a matched donor along with a dose of his own engineered T cells. It was hoped that the T cells would help the patient resist HIV infection of his new bone marrow. If, instead, the engineered T cells caused damage to the patient, they would be destroyed by administering a drug that would cause them to self-destruct. The HyTK gene also enabled researchers to detect whether the T cells were surviving in vivo.[76] This strategy can be classified as a cell therapy rather than as a gene therapy. The genetic engineering really serves as a safety device. The clinical trial of this approach began in February 1993 and is still ongoing.[77]

A different plausible AIDS gene therapy is derived from the infection mechanism of HIV. HIV acts first by binding to certain sites on the surface of cells. These sites are called CD-4 receptors and are encoded by CD-4 genes. Researchers hope to find a mechanism that can deliver CD-4 genes, engineered into *decoy* cells, into patients, thereby luring HIV away from the important immune system cells it usually invades.[78]

Additional approaches involve transducing cells in vitro with genes that could enhance a patient's ability to fight an HIV infection or interfere with the HIV life cycle. When the transduced cells are placed into the patient's body, they should secrete a factor into his or her circulation that will bolster the body's defenses or directly affect HIV. Several strategies designed to directly kill HIV-infected cells or to interfere with HIV's life cycle by inhibiting HIV RNA or HIV proteins are also being tested.[79]

As French Anderson has commented: "HIV is a very clever adversary. It is highly unlikely that any single tactic will work. A combination of several types of attack simultaneously and/or sequentially will probably be needed."[80]

Other Candidate Diseases for the Future

Hemoglobin diseases. Sickle cell anemia and beta-thalassemia are two of several genetic diseases characterized by abnormalities in human hemoglobin, the blood component that is responsible for transporting oxygen. Individuals afflicted with these diseases suffer severe symptoms such as anemia, painful crises, and sometimes death.[81] Early in the development of gene therapy, long before the first human experiment was launched, hemoglobin diseases were considered good candidates for initial gene therapy trials. As knowledge accumulated, however, it became apparent that gene therapy for hemoglobin diseases such as beta-thalassemia and sickle cell disease would be difficult to achieve, because the production of the hemoglobin molecule depends on extraordinarily complex gene regulation.[82] The hemoglobin molecule is comprised of several subunits that must be present in blood cells in delicately balanced amounts. Not only are these subunits produced by several separate genes, but the genes are grouped on two distinct chromosomes.[83] That the healthy human body coordinates the expression of these several genes is nothing short of miraculous. For scientists to understand and mimic that coordination will be no easy matter. And if one added gene's expression is not coordinated with the expression of the other genes that produce subunits, the resulting imbalance itself constitutes a disease state.[84] Therefore, although sickle cell anemia and beta-thalassemia are still posited as potential gene therapy candidates by some, researchers have, for the most part, moved on to other diseases as early candidates for gene therapy. It is possible that recent research results involving retroviral vectors expressing hemoglobin genes in vitro will revive interest in the use of gene therapy for hemoglobin disease treatment.[85]

Muscular dystrophy. Muscular dystrophy is a disease characterized by progressive muscle deterioration, which starts in the lower extremities and steals up the legs, to the hips, the respiratory muscles, and the heart. Muscular dystrophy almost always leads to death by the age of 30. Duchenne muscular dystrophy (DMD), the most common form of this cruel disease, primarily afflicts boys. DMD is caused by a mutation in the dystrophin gene, most often a deletion. For unknown reasons, if the dystrophin protein does not function properly, muscle cell death results. The key behind gene therapy for DMD is the delivery of an error-free copy of the dystrophin gene into the muscle cells of DMD patients.[86]

The dystrophin gene, the largest human gene known, is too large to be delivered to cells via any of the commonly used viral vectors.[87] Similarly, the dystrophin protein is large, complex, and not directly deliverable to cells in its active form. Nevertheless, Dr. Peter Law, formerly of the University of Tennessee,[88] and others have developed a cell-grafting type of method which may prove effective for *indirectly* delivering properly functioning dystrophin genes into patients' cells. This method takes advantage of the peculiar ability of muscle cells to fuse and share proteins.

The proposed treatment, which has worked in mice and is currently being tested in humans, involves injecting healthy muscle cells into the muscles of DMD patients. The healthy cells are obtained from the fathers of the patients and grown in culture in the laboratory before they are administered. It is hoped that these healthy cells will contribute normal dystrophin genes and the normal dystrophin protein to the patients' muscles, thereby preventing their deterioration.[89]

Researchers would like to deliver functioning dystrophin genes directly into the muscle cells of DMD patients. But so far, no one has devised a method for delivering the dystrophin gene into all the muscles of the body.

Ethical Issues

An Initial Question: Is This Kind of Treatment Different?

In the ethical discussions that began in the late 1960s, commentators on human gene therapy sometimes seemed to assume that this technique was qualitatively different from other types of therapeutic interventions. However, as the ethical discussion of gene therapy has progressed, somatic cell gene therapy has increasingly been viewed as a natural and logical *extension* of current techniques for treating disease. Which of these views is correct?

On balance, the gene-therapy-as-extension view seems to be the more appropriate one. There are several reasons for adopting this view. First, because somatic cell gene therapy affects only nonreproductive cells, none of the genetic changes produced by somatic cell gene therapy will be passed on to the patient's children. Second, in some cases the products of the genetically modified somatic cells are similar to medications that patients can take as an alternative treatment. For example, there are enzyme therapies currently available for both ADA deficiency and Gaucher disease, but both enzyme therapies are very expensive and must be administered frequently. Third, some of the techniques currently used in somatic cell gene therapy closely resemble other widely used medical interventions—especially the transplantation of organs or tissues.

Several examples noted in the earlier part of this chapter illustrate how similar at least some somatic cell approaches are to transplantation. In the protocol for treating ADA deficiency, some of the patients' T cells were removed from their bodies and had the missing ADA gene added to them. The genetically modified cells were then returned to the patients' bodies, where they began to produce the missing enzyme, ADA. If the patients involved in this early gene therapy study had had healthy siblings whose cells closely matched their own, the alternative to gene therapy would have been a bone marrow transplant. In effect, the T cells of the healthy sibling (or more technically the stem cells that produce the T cells) would have replaced the patients' own ADA-deficient T cells.

The case is similar with cystic fibrosis (CF). Increasingly, lung transplants are being employed in the treatment of this disease. The cells in the transplanted lung will not have the genetic defect that causes CF and will therefore be able to function normally in the recipient. However, such transplants are expensive and highly invasive procedures, and there is a perpetual shortage of healthy organs for transplantation. Further, because transplanted organs never match the recipient's genotype exactly, except in the case of identical twins, the recipient will likely have to take drugs indefinitely to prevent his or her immune system from rejecting the transplant as foreign tissue. Somatic cell gene therapy seems to many observers to be a less invasive approach than the transplantation of a major organ. In addition, because it is the patient's own cells that are being genetically modified, there is a much lower probability that the cells will be rejected as foreign.

Major Ethical Questions Concerning Gene-Therapy Research

In the review of proposals to perform gene therapy research with human beings, seven questions are central:

1. What is the disease to be treated?
2. What alternative interventions are available for the treatment of this disease?
3. What is the anticipated or potential harm of the experimental gene therapy procedure?
4. What is the anticipated or potential benefit of the experimental gene therapy procedure?
5. What procedure will be followed to ensure fairness in the selection of patient–subjects?
6. What steps will be taken to ensure that patients, or their parents or guardians, give informed and voluntary consent to participating in the research?
7. How will the privacy of patients and the confidentiality of their medical information be protected?

Taken together, questions 1–4 constitute a kind of first hurdle, or initial threshold, that gene therapy research proposals must clear. If these questions are not satisfactorily answered, questions 5–7 will not even need to be asked. However, if the first four questions are satisfactorily answered, and the risk–benefit ratio for the proposed research seems appropriate, questions 5–7 remain as a second hurdle—a set of important procedural safeguards for prospective subjects in the research. (For the full text of the "Points to Consider," see Appendix D.)

What is the disease to be treated? Question 1 asks both a simple and a more profound question. It asks simply for the name of a condition or a disorder that is regarded by reasonable people to be a malfunction in the human body. Thus, "cystic fibrosis" would be an acceptable answer to the first question, while "average height" would not. At a more profound level, question 1 asks whether the disease or condition put forward as an early candidate for somatic cell gene therapy is sufficiently serious or life-threatening to merit being treated with a highly experimental technique. As the list of disorders treated in the first 100 gene therapy studies indicates, the conditions proposed for possible treatment by means of gene therapy do gravely compromise the quality and duration of human life.

It must be acknowledged that two of the disorders included in the above list do not qualify as life-threatening: rheumatoid arthritis and peripheral artery disease. Rheumatoid arthritis is a chronic condition that often causes severe pain to the person who is suffering from it, but this disease alone generally does not cause a patient's death. Similarly, peripheral artery disease in, for example, the lower leg and ankle of a person with diabetes will not cause the patient's death. However, this condition can be limb-threatening. That is, a limb that does not receive a sufficient flow of oxygen may need to be amputated in order to prevent gangrene from developing in the limb. In the future, gene therapy protocols may also be submitted that seek to preserve sight by taking new approaches to the treatment of currently untreatable eye diseases.

Philosophers have argued at considerable length about the precise definitions of health and disease.[90] For our analysis we have adopted a rather standard definition of health, "species-typical functioning."[91] It seems clear that all of the conditions to be treated by the first 100 gene therapy protocols represent significant deviations from the physiological norm of species-typical functioning and therefore qualify as bona fide diseases. But are there reasonable limits to the notion of disease? How far would we will be willing to extend the concept? At the far extremes exemplified in discriminatory social programs both past and present, we would never want to see human characteristics like gender, ethnicity, or skin color regarded as diseases. However, serious mental illness would be included within the scope of our definition. We would not consider mild obesity or a crooked nose or larger-than-average ears to be significant deviations from species-typical functioning. However, serious obesity that threatened to shorten life might well qualify as a disease. In each case a condition will need to be evaluated in the light of species-typical functioning and a judgment will have to be made about the extent to which the condition compromises such functioning.[92]

What alternative interventions are available for the treatment of this disease? Question 2 asks about alternative therapies. If available modes of treatment provide relief from the most serious consequences of a disease without major side effects and at reasonable cost, the disease may not be a good candidate for early clinical trials of gene therapy in humans. For example, phenylketonuria (PKU) is a hereditary disorder that can be detected in newborns through a simple blood test. Dietary therapy suffices to prevent the brain damage that would otherwise occur in children afflicted with the disorder. Therefore, PKU is probably not a good early candidate for gene therapy. Similarly, the harmful effects of diabetes can be controlled quite well in most patients through the use of insulin produced by recombinant DNA techniques. Thus, diabetes may be a later rather than an earlier candidate for gene therapy research.

The determination that an alternative therapy is sufficiently effective is always a judgment call. In the review process for the first ADA deficiency study, it was noted that bone marrow transplantation was an effective treatment for children who had genetically matched siblings and that a synthetic form of ADA was available for use in ADA-deficient patients. The synthetic form of ADA was derived from the ADA produced by cattle and was linked, or conjugated, with the chemical PEG. The proponents of gene therapy for ADA deficiency pointed out that PEG-ADA could stimulate a hostile response by the human immune system because the synthetic compound was derived from cattle and thus might be perceived as foreign. The proponents also noted that, while most ADA-deficient patients benefited somewhat from treatment with PEG-ADA, they were still susceptible to many infections. Further, the high cost of PEG-ADA, about $250,000 per year, put this synthetic treatment out of the reach of most families. Thus, the reviewers of the initial ADA gene therapy protocol ultimately concluded that in families where children had no matched sibling donors, the alternative therapy of PEG-ADA was not wholly satisfactory. There was therefore space or justification for the development of gene therapy as a possibly superior approach to the treatment of this life-threatening pediatric disease.

As the field of gene therapy matures, the requirement that there be no effective alternative therapy may need to be relaxed. At some point there will need to be well-controlled studies that compare the gene therapy approach with alternative approaches to treatment of the same disease. However, given the novelty of gene therapy in 1990 and the uncertainty about its potential benefits and harms, it seems to us to have been appropriate to limit the earliest gene therapy trials to diseases and groups of patients for whom no alternative therapies were available.

What is the anticipated or potential harm of the experimental gene-therapy procedure? Question 3 concerns the anticipated or possible harm of somatic cell gene therapy. In responding to this question, researchers are asked to base their statements on the best available *data* from preclinical studies in vitro or in laboratory animal models like mice or monkeys. The use of domesticated (technically, replication-deficient) viruses as vectors in many somatic-cell gene-therapy studies raises one important safety question: How certain can researchers be that the domesticated viruses will not regain the genes that have been removed from them and thus regain the capacity to reproduce and cause an infection in the patient? A second kind of safety question arises from the "unguided-missile" quality of retroviral vectors. As noted earlier in this chapter, researchers cannot predict where a retroviral vector with its attached gene and marker will "land" within the nucleus of a target cell. It is possible that the vector will integrate into the middle of a gene that is essential to the functioning of the cell and will therefore kill the cell. A further concern is the theoretical possibility that a retroviral vector might integrate beside a quiescent oncogene (cancer-causing gene) and stimulate it into becoming active. If so, a previously healthy cell might begin to divide uncontrollably and even start a cancer in a particular site. Because of these concerns about risk and safety, researchers are asked to provide data about preclinical studies in animals that, insofar as possible, exactly duplicate the gene therapy studies that they propose to do in human subjects.

What is the anticipated or potential benefit of the experimental gene therapy procedure? The fourth question is in many ways the mirror image of the third. It asks researchers once again to provide data from preclinical studies, but in this case the data should indicate that there is a reasonable expectation of benefit to human patients from their participation in the gene therapy study. One step in the review process for the first approved human-gene therapy study in 1990 illustrates the importance of this point. Drs. Blaese and Anderson had provided impressive safety data to the RAC (the Recombinant DNA Advisory Committee—established in 1974 by NIH; discussed in historical context in Chapter 5) based on their long-term studies in mice and monkeys. However, RAC members were not convinced that the genetic modification of ADA-deficient T cells would be beneficial to human patients. What if the T cells died off quickly, or what if they were overwhelmed by the patients' own ADA-deficient T cells? Fortunately there was a researcher in Milan, Italy, Dr. Claudio Bordignon, who was willing to speak to the RAC about his own research in mice that had an immune deficiency similar to the one that afflicts ADA-deficient human patients. In these animals Dr. Bordignon was able to show that *human* T cells that carry a functioning ADA gene survive longer than ADA-deficient T cells. This was the information that the RAC was seeking, and Dr. Bordignon's report helped to ensure the approval of the Blaese–Anderson proposal.

There has been considerable debate about the appropriate relationship between question 3 and question 4—or between anticipated harm and anticipated benefit of a gene therapy study. Some researchers have argued that if a gene therapy study is not likely to make patients worse off, it should be approved even if the probability of benefit is very low. This rationale may have been the basis for the controversial approval of a gene therapy protocol by former NIH director Bernadine Healy in December 1992. The proposal to treat a single cancer patient had not gone through regular view by the NIH RAC, and there was, in the opinion of most experts, little probability that it would benefit the terminally ill patient. Nonetheless, Dr. Healy approved the protocol on a "compassionate use" basis.[93] Since late 1992 the RAC has further discussed the requisite harm–benefit ratio in gene therapy studies. A majority of the committee members seem to have adopted the following view: Even if a gene therapy protocol provides a satisfactory answer to question 3 (about harm), it must also offer at least a low probability of benefit to the patients who are invited to enter the protocol, *and* it must have an excellent scientific design, so that the information gathered from studying the early patients will be useful to later patients and to the entire field of gene therapy research. That is, there must also be a satisfactory answer to question 4.

If these first four questions are satisfactorily answered, researchers have cleared a first hurdle or crossed an important threshold. They have demonstrated that the ratio of probable benefit to probable harm in a proposed study is sufficiently positive to justify proceeding to research in human beings. The remaining three questions ask how the research will be done, or, in other words, outline procedural safeguards for the patients who will be invited to take part in the gene therapy studies.

What procedure will be followed to ensure fairness in the selection of patient–subjects? The first of the procedural questions, and the fifth question overall, asks how patients will be selected in a fair manner. With very rare disorders, like familial hypercholesterolemia and ADA deficiency, fairness in the selection process was relatively unproblematic. Virtually every patient with the condition who was not too ill to participate was considered a candidate for gene therapy and invited to enroll in the studies. However, when somatic cell gene therapy began to be used for more prevalent conditions like brain tumors, the selection process became much more difficult. For example, the first study of gene therapy for brain tumors was led by Edward Oldfield and Kenneth Culver at the National Institutes of Health. Their proposal was initially approved for the study of 20 patients. Within the first year of their study the offices of Drs. Oldfield and Culver received more than 1,000 inquiries by patients, their family members and friends, and even governors and legislators. It was therefore quite important that a fair procedure, like first-come first-served, be in place to use in selecting among the many candidates for treatment.

In the review of the first 100 gene therapy protocols two other questions of fairness in selecting subjects have also arisen. The first question is whether children should be included in the initial studies, assuming that some children do survive to adulthood with the disease. The first gene therapy study, for severe combined immune deficiency (SCID), involved children precisely because, until now, almost no children with this disorder live to complete their teenage years. However, some patients with familial hypercholesterolemia do live to be 30, as do an increasing number of cystic fibrosis (CF) patients. There are two opposing ethical perspectives on the involvement of children in the early stages of clinical trials. The classical position, formulated in the early 1970s in the United States, was that clinical trials should be completed in adults first, before children are exposed to the potential harms of such trials.[94] The revisionist position of the late 1980s and 1990s is that participants in clinical trials are carefully monitored and that they often are the first people in a society to have access to new and possibly effective treatments. Therefore no class of individuals, whether women or members of ethnic minorities or children, should be excluded from the potential benefits of timely participation in clinical trials.[95]

A second question is closely related to the alternative-therapy question discussed above. It concerns the stage of disease at which people with serious disease should receive gene therapy. Already in 1987, during the review of the "Preclinical Data Document," there had been vigorous debate about whether gene therapy should be regarded as last-ditch therapy. In the early studies of gene therapy, patients had generally not been helped by alternative therapies, or no alternative therapies were available. As the field has matured, and as researchers have gained more confidence in the safety of gene therapy (if not in its effectiveness), the question has increasingly been raised, "Why not employ gene therapy at earlier stages in the disease process where it might have a better chance to prevent the deterioration of the patient's condition?"

What steps will be taken to ensure that patients, or their parents or guardians, give informed and voluntary consent to participating in the research? The next procedural question, and the sixth question overall, concerns the voluntary and informed consent of patients or, in the case of minors, of their parents or guardians. It is always a challenge for researchers to convey to potential patient–subjects the important facts about their disease or condition, the major alternative treatments, and the precise procedures to be followed in the research. With a cutting-edge technology like human gene therapy this generic problem becomes even more difficult. For gene therapy studies, patients or their parents or guardians will frequently need a short course on how recombinant DNA research is conducted, how vectors are constructed, what cell types are targeted, how genes are inserted into cells, and how genes function in cells. In the case of specific gene therapy studies, additional modules may have to be added to the short course. For example, in the case of gene therapy for SCID, patients or their parents or guardians will need additional information on the human immune system and how specific kinds of cells, like T cells, function. While this educational responsibility may initially seem daunting, the question about voluntary, informed consent simply points to the importance of an extensive and ongoing dialogue between researchers and subjects, rather than the momentary act of signing a multiple-page consent form.

The response of researchers to question 6 has varied considerably. Some gene therapy proposals have included detailed information, including charts that outline the sequence and timing of proposed procedures, for patients. Other written consent forms have been woefully incomplete or have included ambiguous wording about who pays for procedures required by the research or about how the sponsoring institution deals with patients who are accidentally injured while they participate in research. Further, no external observers are present to monitor the quality of the consent *process* as patients are invited to take part in gene therapy studies. All that can be said with certainty is that the RAC has provided detailed guidance to researchers about the major points that RAC members think should be included in consent forms and that the consent forms themselves are reviewed in a public forum by peers who are not employees of the sponsoring institutions.

How will the privacy of patients and the confidentiality of their medical information be protected? The third procedural question, and the seventh question overall, concerns privacy and confidentiality. There is no single "correct" answer to this question. It merely asks researchers to think through in advance how they and the subjects participating in gene therapy studies will deal with inquiries from the press and the general public. A particular concern was that patients have sufficient privacy and rest following their treatment to allow them "space" to benefit from this experimental approach to treatment. Different researchers and families have adopted varying policies regarding privacy and confidentiality. In the case of the ADA-deficiency protocol, the first two young women treated remained relatively anonymous until the second anniversary (in September 1992) of the first child's initial treatment. Less than a year later, the two children were featured, named, and pictured in a *Time* magazine story.[96] In contrast, the parents of two newborns treated at birth (in a modification of the same protocol) by a different technique using stem cells from umbilical cord blood allowed their names and pictures, and the names and pictures of their infants, to be disclosed almost immediately.[97] Similarly, the first patient in the study that aims to treat peripheral artery disease was interviewed by a reporter for the *New York Times* before he received his first gene transfer.[98]

This final question was included in the "Points to Consider" not to prescribe or proscribe any particular actions by patients or researchers but simply to encourage all parties involved in gene therapy studies to think through, in advance, a strategy for dealing with the press and the media. There had, in fact, been veritable media circuses when several earlier biomedical technologies had first been introduced. One thinks, for example, of the earliest heart transplant recipients, of Barney Clark and his artificial heart, of Baby Fae and her baboon heart, and of Louise Brown, the first "test tube baby." In general, the introduction of gene therapy has been, in our view, more respectful of patients and their families.

Public Attitudes and Expert Opinion about Somatic Cell Gene Therapy

The social context in which somatic-cell gene-therapy research occurs includes the response of both the general public and people who might be called "experts" to the concept as well as the practice of gene therapy. From the 1980s to the present we have a rather detailed record of both public attitudes in the United States and international expert opinion.

The Louis Harris polling organization has taken two snapshots of public attitudes toward gene therapy in the United States. The first survey, conducted by telephone between October 30th and November 17th, 1986, was commissioned by the Congressional Office of Technology Assessment (OTA).[99] In this initial survey, 1,273 telephone interviews were completed, and the sampling error was in the range of plus or minus 2–3%. The second survey, conducted by phone between April 17th and April 30th, 1992, was commissioned by the March of Dimes Birth Defects Foundation.[100] In this second survey a national cross section of 1,000 adults were interviewed, and the sampling error was plus or minus 3%.

Public knowledge of "genetic engineering" (1986) and "gene therapy" (1992) seems to be surprisingly meager. In answer to the 1986 question, "How much have you heard or read about genetic engineering?" in 1986, 24% of respondents said, "Almost nothing," and another 39% replied, "Relatively little."[101] Despite rather extensive news coverage of the initial gene therapy experiments in the intervening years, the 1992 survey discovered similar levels of professed ignorance. The 1992 question was, "How much have you heard or read about gene therapy?" Sixty percent of respondents said, "Almost nothing," and another 26% acknowledged that they had heard or read "Relatively little."[102]

Despite their lack of knowledge the telephone respondents in the two surveys proceeded to answer the remaining questions put to them by the interviewers. The respondents' general attitudes about the ethics of human gene therapy were elicited with rather different questions in 1986 and 1992. In the OTA survey of 1986 the question and response were as shown in Table 2-1.

In the 1992 survey, the corresponding question was much more positively phrased and included the assumption that the gene therapy procedure would be safe. Not surprisingly, the response was also much more positive (Table 2-2).

Another way of assessing public attitudes toward gene therapy is to ask whether

Table 2-1. The Morality of Human Cell Manipulation

Some people believe that genetic alteration of human cells to treat disease is simply another form of medical treatment. Other people believe that changing the genetic makeup of human cells is morally wrong, regardless of the purpose. On balance, do you feel that changing the genetic makeup of human cells is morally wrong, or not?[103]

	Morally Wrong	Not Morally Wrong	Not Sure
Total (1,273)	42%	52%	6%

Table 2-2. General Attitude About Gene Therapy

If it were safe, would you strongly approve, somewhat approve, somewhat disapprove, or strongly disapprove of gene therapy to treat or cure genetic diseases?[104]

Strongly Approve	Somewhat Approve	Somewhat Disapprove	Strongly Disapprove	Not Sure
47%	41%	4%	4%	4%

people would be willing to make use of this new technique for themselves or one of their children. Tables 2-3 and 2-4 provide the responses to identical questions asked by the Louis Harris organization in 1986 and 1992 (1986 data in parentheses).

Two specific scenarios for somatic cell gene therapy were presented to the respondents in the 1986 and 1992 surveys. The word "genetic" was dropped from the first scenario in 1992, perhaps in part because multiple gene-therapy proposals for treating cancers had been developed in the meantime. Otherwise the two scenarios were identical.

One final way to assess public attitudes toward somatic cell gene therapy is to inquire whether members of the public think that research in this arena should be continued or stopped. In the 1986 survey only a general question had been asked about whether "research into genetic engineering should be continued or should be stopped." Eighty-two percent of respondents replied, "Continued," while 13%

Table 2-3. Willingness to Undergo Gene Therapy

If tests showed that you were likely to get a serious or fatal genetic disease late in life, how willing would you be to have those genes corrected before symptoms appear—very willing, somewhat willing, somewhat unwilling, very unwilling?[105]

Very Willing	Somewhat Willing	Somewhat Unwilling	Very Unwilling	Not Sure
30% (35)	49% (43)	10% (12)	9% (9)	2% (2)

1992 vs. (1986).

Table 2-4. Willingness to Have a Child Undergo Gene Therapy

If you had a child with a usually fatal genetic disease, how willing would you be to have the child undergo therapy to have those genes corrected—very willing, somewhat willing, somewhat unwilling, very unwilling?[106]

Very Willing	Somewhat Willing	Somewhat Unwilling	Very Unwilling	Not Sure
52% (51)	36% (35)	5% (7)	4% (4)	3% (3)

1992 vs. (1986)

said, "Stopped."[107] The 1992 survey asked more specifically whether "research into gene therapy should be continued or should be stopped." Eighty-nine percent of respondents favored continuation, while only 8% advocated the cessation of this line of research.[108]

What is the importance for ethical analysis of these ethical judgments by a random sample of the U.S. public? There is certainly no easy or automatic leap from the fact that a majority of the general public think that something is the case to its actually being the case—either in ethics or in science. In the realm of ethics, prejudice or bias sometimes interferes with making correct judgments. Think, for example, about traditional biases against members of various ethnic or racial groups, or about 19th-century majority views regarding voting rights for women. On the other hand, the moral judgments of the general public, as reflected in survey data, can be relevant in several ways. First, if people understand at least in a general way the questions they are answering, their judgments reflect a kind of common morality.[109] Thus, it seems clear from the survey data that a majority of the public is open to the use of genetic technology in the war against disease and has not been frightened into opposing genetic technology in principle by social critics like Jeremy Rifkin. Further, the more urgent the medical situation, the more likely respondents are to approve the use of gene therapy in the attempt to rem-

Table 2-5. Opinions about Specific Applications of Human Cell Manipulation

How do you feel about scientists changing the makeup of human cells to cure a usually fatal [genetic] disease? To reduce the risk of developing a fatal disease later in life? Would you strongly approve, somewhat approve, somewhat disapprove, or strongly disapprove?

	Strongly Approve	Somewhat Approve	Somewhat Disapprove	Strongly Disapprove	Not Sure
Cure a usually fatal [genetic] disease?	57% (48)	30% (35)	5% (7)	7% (7)	1% (2)
Reduce the risk of developing a fatal disease later in life?	41% (39)	37% (38)	11% (12)	8% (9)	3% (2)

1992 vs. (1986).

edy the situation. The survey data also reveal a surprising willingness of the general public to consider gene therapy for themselves or their children—despite their admitted lack of knowledge on the topic. Finally, the poll data reflect strong support for research on gene therapy as one possible means for combating disease.

Second, data from polls like the two Harris surveys cited can serve as a salutary check on the rhetoric of politicians and public commentators. Any public figure who asserted, "The overwhelming majority of the American people oppose genetic engineering," could now be challenged to define what he or she meant by the term *genetic engineering*. If the answer were, "Any method of changing genes," the public figure could be asked about the specific techniques of gene addition currently being employed in somatic cell gene therapy. The results of the two Harris surveys could also be adduced, and the public figure could be asked whether he or she had any evidence from other public-opinion polls. In short, pubic opinion and its reflection in surveys can help to raise the level of public discourse about important questions that are facing a society.

For international public opinion, similar surveys do not currently exist except for Japan and New Zealand.[110] However, beginning in 1980, numerous expert committees, commissions, and spokespeople for major religious groups have published policy positions on the ethics of human gene therapy. We have identified 28 policy statements on this topic from the years 1980 through 1993 (Table 2-6).

These 28 policy statements represent multiple professions, religious traditions, and cultures, including most advanced industrialized countries. Yet on somatic cell gene therapy a remarkable consensus emerges from the statements: All 28 agree that somatic cell gene therapy for the cure of serious disease is ethically acceptable in principle. There are few issues in all of biomedical ethics on which one would be able to discover such unanimous agreement!

Again in the case of the policy statements by experts there remains a nagging question. What is the importance for ethical analysis of the ethical judgments of experts from various fields? There is, of course, the possibility that various individuals and groups will read previous statements and merely follow, in lemming-like fashion, what their predecessors have said. In addition, the so-called experts may all be recruited from one academic field or area or from one social class and therefore may exhibit a systematic bias. However, on other issues in bioethics— like surrogate motherhood, for example—there are clear differences of opinion among experts in different countries and cultures.[111] Thus, a unanimous consensus of the 28 policy statements by representatives of multiple academic and professional fields suggests at least a measure of cross-cultural agreement on an important issue. To be sure, this consensus of the experts on the ethical acceptability of somatic cell gene therapy provides no guarantee that this practice is in fact ethically acceptable. However, ethical judgements do not allow for mathematical precision. In our judgment, we are less likely to make a serious moral mistake

Table 2-6. Policy Statements on Human Gene Therapy: An International Chronology

1980

World Council of Churches, Conference on Faith, Science, and the Future, *Faith and Science in an Unjust World*

1982

Parliamentary Assembly, Council of Europe: Recommendation 934 (1982) on genetic engineering

World Council of Churches, Working Committee on Church and Society, *Manipulating Life*

United States, President's Commission for the Study of Ethical Problems in Medicine and Biomedical Research, *Splicing Life* report

1983

Pope John Paul II, Address on "The Ethics of Genetic Manipulation" to the 35th General Assembly of the World Medical Association in Venice

1984

Denmark, Indenrigsministeriet (Ministry of the Interior) *Fremskridtets Pris* (*The Price of Progress*)

Sweden, Gen-Ethikkommittén (Genetic Ethics Committee), *Genetisk Integritet* (*Genetic Integrity*)

U.S., Congress, Office of Technology Assessment, *Human Gene Therapy: Background Paper*

1985

U.S., National Institutes of Health, Human Gene Therapy Subcommittee (formerly, Working Group on Human Gene Therapy), "Points to Consider in the Design and Submission of Human Somatic-Cell Gene Therapy Protocols"

Federal Republic of Germany, Justice Minister and Minister for Research and Technology, Working Group (the Benda Commission), *In-Vitro Fertilisation, Genomanalyse und Gentherapie* (*In Vitro Fertilization, Genome-Analysis, and Gene Therapy*)

1986

National Council of Churches, Governing Board, policy statement on "Genetic Science for Human Benefit"

1987

German Federal Republic, Tenth Bundestag, Enquete-Kommission (Committee of Inquiry), *Chancen und Risiken der Gentechnologie* (*Opportunities and Risks of Genetic Technology*)

World Medical Association, "Statement on Genetic Counseling and Genetic Engineering" (39th World Medical Assembly, Madrid)

Canada, Medical Research Council, *Guidelines on Research Involving Human Subjects*

Australia, National Health and Medical Research Council, Medical Research Ethics Committee, *Ethical Aspects of Research on Human Gene Therapy*

1988

European Medical Research Councils, "Gene Therapy in Man"

American Medical Association, Council on Ethical and Judicial Affairs, "Opinion on Gene Therapy and Surrogate Mothers" [Report E: (I-88); title provided]

Switzerland, Commission d'Experts pour la Génétique Humaine et la Médecine de la Reproduction, *Rapport* (*The Amstad-Report*)

Continued

Table 2–6. Continued

1989	
	Canada, Medical Research Council, *Discussion Paper: Research on Gene Therapy in Humans: Background and Guidelines*
	European Commission, Working Party, *Ethics of New Reproductive Technologies* (*The Glover Report*)
	World Council of Churches, Subunit on Church and Society, *Biotechnology: Its Challenge to the Churches and the World*
	Netherlands, Dutch Health Council, Committee, *Heredity: Science and Society: On the Possibilities and Limits of Genetic Testing and Gene Therapy*
1990	
	Council for International Organizations of Medical Sciences (CIOMS), "Genetics, Ethics and Human Values: Human Genome Mapping, Genetic Screening and Gene Therapy (The "Declaration of Inuyama")
	Canada, Medical Research Council, *Guidelines for Research on Somatic Cell Gene Therapy in Humans*
	France, Comité Consultatif National d'Ethique pour les Sciences de la Vie et de la Santé, *Avis sur la Thérapie Génique* (*Opinion on Gene Therapy*)
1991	
	Norway, Ministry of Health and Social Affairs, Ethics Committee, *Man and Biotechnology*
1992	
	United Kingdom, Committee on the Ethics of Human Gene Therapy [the Clothier committee], *Report*
1993	
	Canada, Royal Commission on New Reproductive Technologies, "Gene Therapy and Genetic Alteration," Chapter 29 in *Proceed with Care: Final Report*

if we are guided in our ethical analysis, at least in part, by the consensus view of the experts.[112]

Other Major Questions about Gene Therapy

In addition to the seven questions raised about gene therapy by the "Points to Consider," there are important questions about the current system for conducting and overseeing gene therapy, both in the United States and abroad. The following section of this chapter attempts to step back from the specifics of the first 100 U.S. gene therapy protocols to examine some of these broader issues.

Was gene therapy attempted in patients too soon? This first question asks whether more laboratory research in cell cultures and in animal models should have preceded the first clinical studies with gene therapy. Some critics of current practice have noted that the available vectors for delivering genes to cells are relatively primitive. Other critics argue that basic research on how stem cells work and how they can be modified may facilitate new approaches to gene therapy. A third line of criticism is that, while a few protocols submitted by researchers for review by the NIH RAC have represented excellent science, many of the protocols have been unoriginal and probably would not have been funded by NIH if the protocols had been reviewed according to the stringent standards of the usual NIH grant application process.

What can be said in response to these criticisms? First, the first somatic-cell gene-therapy studies in human beings were preceded by almost 20 years of public discussion and debate.[113] Even the initial protocol, approved in 1990, had been debated in near-final form from 1987 through early 1990. Thus, the introduction of gene therapy as a new biomedical technology has been more deliberate and more cautious than the first use of several other important techniques—for example, genetic screening for PKU in newborns, heart transplantation, and test tube (in vitro) fertilization. Second, even though the currently published evidence is sparse, there is at least a suggestion of clinical benefit in the initial gene therapy study for patients with SCID. At the same time, however, it must be acknowledged that the level of success in the first 60–70 gene therapy studies in the United States has been disappointing even to the technique's strongest advocates. In part because of this disappointment, the NIH director, Harold Varmus, recently asked an expert committee to review the NIH investment in gene therapy.[114]

Which diseases are the best early candidates for gene therapy? We have seen in this chapter what the target diseases are in the first 100 U.S. gene therapy protocols. Are various types of cancers sufficiently important to merit having more than 60% of the protocols directed toward cancer? Is 22 of the first 100 studies the appropriate share for the thousands of genetic diseases? And do HIV infection and AIDS deserve more or less than 12% of the research effort?

The answers to these questions, like the answers to many resource allocation questions, stretch human knowledge and judgment to their limits. One approach to answering the questions is to ask: What is the burden of disease, in terms of premature death, suffering, lost work, and disability, caused by each disorder? The answer to this question provides at least one dimension of the answer to the larger question, although it should be noted that the comparison of death, permanent disability, pain and suffering, and temporary disability involves a series of value judgments.[115] However, the burden caused by a certain disease is only part of the picture. There must also be a genuine research opportunity. That is, enough progress in understanding and perhaps even in treating a disease must have been made to allow a next step to have a reasonable hope of succeeding. In the case of SCID, a very rare genetic disorder, one feature that made the disease a good early candidate for gene therapy studies was that it had been cured through bone marrow transplants from matched sibling donors. Thus, researchers had good leads in their quest to treat the disease in children who lacked such donors. Further, the gene for ADA had been isolated in the laboratory and was available for clinical use. One other safety feature for SCID was that the gene did not have to be carefully regulated. An overproduction of ADA by a turned-on gene would not, it seemed, harm the recipient patient. For these reasons SCID appeared to be an excellent early candidate for gene therapy, even though it is a rare disorder with a rather small national disease burden.

For the future the expert committee appointed by the NIH director may have some suggestions about an overall strategy for setting priorities among diseases, particularly if one or two diseases seem to have received inordinate attention thus far. On the other hand, centralized planning and long-term strategies may also have their pitfalls. There is much to be said for allowing considerable latitude to researchers in choosing the diseases that they consider to be plausible early candidates for gene therapy and in developing creative new approaches to the experimental treatment of those diseases. One of the most intriguing aspects of science is the factor of serendipity. One never knows in advance which scientists, which laboratory, which topic, and which approach will produce the next breakthrough, with unexpected benefits in a wide variety of seemingly unrelated fields.

To what extent should commercial considerations drive the selection of target diseases? This question is closely related to the preceding question. It is not surprising that, with the increasing involvement of private industry in somatic cell gene therapy there has also been a increasing focus on diseases that are prevalent in the United States. The largest trials to date, in terms of the numbers of patients, are studies directed toward HIV infection and AIDS. As noted earlier, cancers of various types are the targets in almost two-thirds of the first 100 protocols. And among genetic diseases cystic fibrosis, the most prevalent genetic disorder among Caucasians, commands the most attention.

We should not be surprised that commercial firms would look, first and foremost, at larger rather than smaller markets. If gene therapy proves to be a successful strategy, these firms will one day provide the bridge from the laboratory to large numbers of patients. At the same time, however, there are the so-called *orphan diseases*, which strike people in numbers too small to provide a strong incentive for an investment in research. There are, again, no easy solutions to this general problem in the U.S. health care system. Public investment in research is no doubt one part of the solution: NIH researchers and researchers supported by federal funds have the option of targeting diseases that affect relatively few people. Success in treating rare diseases may, in turn, provide clues that will assist in the treatment of more prevalent diseases. However, by far the most important part of the solution to the problem of gene therapy for rare disorders will have to await major reform in the health care system.

How is national oversight for gene therapy working? Virtually all U.S. gene therapy proposals go through a national public review process at the National Institutes of Health. Under a new consolidated review process with the Food and Drug Administration (FDA), only proposals that raise novel issues are reviewed publicly at quarterly RAC meetings. For the other proposals, basic information about the researchers, the title of the protocol, the target cell, the vectors, and the sponsors is made available in a public summary. All serious adverse events experienced by patients are also reported at each quarterly RAC meeting. In addition, at periodic intervals—annually in the future—a public report on virtually all U.S. gene therapy studies is compiled and presented at a public RAC meeting. This report allows any interested person to learn the most important facts, except for the effectiveness of treatment, about ongoing and already-closed clinical trials of gene therapy. For example, one can find out how many patients are enrolled in each trial and how many adverse effects have occurred. If the results of a study have been published, the publication is cited.

One of the authors of this book has been much too closely involved with the public review process for gene therapy to be objective in judging it. However, several comments are in order. The level of public accountability that has existed for the early stages of gene therapy research is unprecedented in the history of clinical research. In fact, the NIH RAC has functioned as a kind of national research ethics committee (or institutional review board) for one new biomedical technology, gene therapy. Further, the RAC review process has provided a model for several other countries as they have established their own national review committees for gene therapy. In most cases the parallel committees in other nations do not meet in public, but their members often attend RAC meetings and sometimes report that RAC deliberations are helpful to them in evaluating protocols that come before them in their confidential review process.

Some U.S. commercial firms and some university researchers have found dual review to be burdensome and have campaigned to have the FDA provide the sole review for gene therapy studies. They argue that, even if the RAC was needed in the early 1990s for the earliest gene therapy studies, it has now outlived its usefulness. Our own view as authors is that the public review of selected protocols and the periodic reports on the current status of gene therapy are still important to the U.S. public, to the press and the media, and to members of the United States Congress. Public review and regular monitoring are essential to public accountability, in our view.

To what extent are researchers in other countries involved in gene therapy research? We have focused primarily on gene therapy in the United States because more studies have been initiated here than in any other nation. However, gene therapy research is proceeding in the United Kingdom, France, the Netherlands, Germany, Italy, Japan, and China—and in perhaps other nations as well.

For the most part, the studies that have been made public parallel those that are being conducted in the United States. For example, SCID is the target disease in several countries. A study for which there is no parallel is the Chinese protocol that seeks to treat hemophilia B.[116]

How useful will somatic cell gene therapy be in the long run? The honest answer to this final question is, "It's too early to know the answer to this question with any degree of certainty."

Some critics of gene therapy have argued that the future does not look bright for this approach to treatment. They note that, using current techniques, gene therapy probably costs at least $100,000 per year per patient, with ongoing retreatment and monitoring being required for all patients. They also assert, quite rightly, that alternative treatments, like drug treatment for people with cystic fibrosis, are also improving and may ultimately make gene therapy unnecessary.

So long as gene therapy requires repeated treatments by very specialized laboratories that can introduce genes into target cells by means of engineered viral vectors, gene therapy will remain a relatively expensive approach to the treatment of disease. It will, under these conditions, be of very limited utility in the war on human disease. There are visionaries, however, who foresee at least the possibility that the gene therapy approach may become as routine and pervasive as current techniques like the use of immunizations or antibiotics. W. French Anderson, for example, dreams of a day when a "magic bullet" will be available that would "enable healing genes to enter the bloodstream and go directly to the cell that needs help."[117] In the words of Anderson, "I'd like to go to Africa with 10,000 vials and inject the gene to cure sickle-cell anemia."[118]

Notes

1. Larry Thompson, "Human Gene Therapy Test Working," *Washington Post*, December 16, 1990, p. A6; Natalie Angier, "Doctors Have Success Treating a Blood Disease by Altering Genes," *New York Times*, July 28, 1991, Section I, p. 20.

2. Experimental protocol submitted to the Human Gene Therapy Subcommittee of the Recombinant DNA Advisory Committee, entitled "Treatment of Severe Combined Immunodeficiency Disease (SCID) due to Adenosine Deaminase (ADA) Deficiency with Autologous Lymphocytes Transduced with a Human ADA Gene," pp. 2–3.

3. Ibid., p. 3.

4. Eve K. Nichols, *Human Gene Therapy* (Cambridge, MA: Harvard University Press, 1988), p. 217.

5. Response to Points to Consider for ADA Deficiency protocol, p. 15.

6. Thomas D. Gelehrter and Francis S. Collins, *Principles of Medical Genetics* (Baltimore: Williams & Wilkins, 1990), p. 295; Natalie Angier, "New Genetic Treatment Given Vote of Confidence," *New York Times*, June 3, 1990, Section I, p. 25.

7. Response to Points to Consider, p. 13 (22).

8. W. French Anderson, "Prospects for Human Gene Therapy," *Science* 226(4673): 402; 26 October 1984; John E. Dick, "Retrovirus-Mediated Gene Transfer into Hemato-

poietic Stem Cells," *Annals of the New York Academy of Sciences* 507: 242–251; 1987. Shortly after the human ADA gene therapy experiment achieved success, the U.S. Patent and Trademark Office granted a patent to Stanford University molecular biologist Irving Weissman and colleagues at SyStemix, a biotechnology company, for their process for isolating stem cells and for the isolated stem cells themselves. See Beverly Merz, "Researchers Find Stem Cell; Clinical Possibilities Touted," *American Medical News*, November 25, 1991, p. 2.

9. Angier, "Doctors Have Success," (note 1); experimental protocol (note 2), p. 24 (59).

10. Response to Points to Consider (note 5), p. 12 (21).

11. R. Michael Blaese, et al., "T Lymphocyte-Directed Gene Therapy for ADA⁻ SCID: Initial Trial Results after 4 Years," *Science* 270(5235): 475–480; 20 October 1995.

12. Ibid., p. 479.

13. Ibid., pp. 475–476.

14. Ibid., p. 477.

15. Ibid., p. 478. For more detailed accounts of this initial gene therapy study in the United States, see Larry Thompson, *Correcting the Code: Inventing the Genetic Cure for the Human Body* (New York: Simon and Schuster, 1994), and Jeff Lyon and Peter Gorner, *Altered Fates: Gene Therapy and the Retooling of Human Life* (New York: W. W. Norton & Company, 1995). For an excellent survey of the status of somatic cell gene therapy in 1995 see Ronald G. Crystal, "Transfer of Genes to Humans: Early Lessons and Obstacles to Success," *Science* 270(5235): 404–410; 20 October 1995.

16. Claudio Bordignon, et al., "Gene Therapy in Peripheral Blood Lymphocytes and Bone Marrow for ADA-Immunodeficient Patients," *Science* 270(5235): 470–475; 20 October 1995.

17. Ibid., pp. 473–474.

18. Gina Kolata, *New York Times*, October 20, 1995, p. A22.

19. A few weeks before the two *Science* articles on gene therapy were published, a newborn substudy of the Blaese–Anderson protocol reported initial results in the treatment of three newborn infants. According to the authors, the genetic modification of CD34+ cells in the umbilical cord blood of three ADA-deficient newborns had resulted in the persistence of the introduced gene in leukocytes (white blood cells) from bone marrow and peripheral blood for 18 months after the initial treatment. All three patients are also receiving PEG-ADA, although the dosages have been reduced. No clinical effects of the genetic modification were expected or observed at the time the article was published. See Donald B. Kohn, et al., "Engraftment of Gene-Modified Umbilical Cord Blood Cells in Neonates with Adenosine Deaminase Deficiency," *Nature Medicine* 1(10): 1017–1023; October 1995.

20. David Baltimore, "Case Analysis 5. Genetic Engineering: the Future—Potential Uses," in National Academy of Sciences, *Research with Recombinant DNA: An Academy Forum, March 7–9, 1977* (Washington, DC: the Academy, 1977), pp. 237–240.

21. W. French Anderson, et al., *Human Gene Therapy: Preclinical Data Document*, submitted to Human Gene Therapy Subcommittee, Recombinant DNA Advisory Committee, on April 24, 1987.

22. Robert C. King and William D. Stansfield, *A Dictionary of Genetics* (4th ed.; New York: Oxford University Press, 1990), p. 276; Thomas D. Gelehrter and Francis S. Collins, *Principles of Medical Genetics* (Baltimore: Williams & Wilkins, 1990), p. 88.

23. King and Stansfield, p. 133.

24. The genomic structure described applies primarily to the type C leukemia viruses. Other retroviruses, such as the lentiviruses (HIV, for example), have a more complicated genomic structure.

25. H. von Melchner and K. Höffken, "Retrovirus Mediated Gene Transfer into Hemopoietic Cells," *Blut* 57(1): 1–5; July 1988; D.A. Williams, "Gene Transfer and Prospects for Somatic Gene Therapy," *Hematology/Oncology Clinics of North America* 2(2): 277–287; June 1988; Dick, op. cit. (note 8); and Maxine Singer and Paul Berg, *Genes and Genomes: A Changing Perspective* (Mill Valley, CA: University Science Books, 1991), pp. 310–311.

26. Singer and Berg, op. cit.

27. Singer and Berg, op. cit.

28. Singer and Berg, op. cit.

29. Personal communication from James Barrett, Genetic Therapy, Inc., May 24, 1996.

30. Oral presentation to the NIH Committee on the Investment in Human Gene Therapy, May 15, 1995.

31. Michael Waldholz, "Genetic Therapy Wins Patent for Use of Gene Treatment," *Wall Street Journal*, March 22, 1995, p. B6; and Teresa Riordan, "A Biotech Company Is Granted Broad Patent and Stock Jumps," *New York Times*, March 22, 1995, p. D1.

32. Carol Ezzell, "Gene Therapy for Rare Cholesterol Disorder," *Science News* 140(15):230; 12 October 1991.

33. Interview with James M. Wilson, October 29, 1991.

34. Interview with James M. Wilson, October 29, 1991; Mariann Grossman et al., "Successful ex vivo Gene Therapy Directed to Liver in a Patient with Familial Hypercholesterolemia," *Nature Genetics* 6(4): 335–341; April 1994. See the comments on this paper in *Nature Genetics* 7(3): 349–350; July 1994.

35. Grossman et al., op. cit.

36. Interview with James S. Wilson, October 29, 1991.

37. Interview with James S. Wilson, October 29, 1991. See also the following report from Wilson's research group: Karen F. Kozarsky et al., "In Vivo Correction of Low Density Lipoprotein Receptor Deficiency in the Watanabe Heritable Hyperlipidemic Rabbit with Recombinant Adenoviruses," *Journal of Biological Chemistry* 269(18): 13695–13702; 6 May 1994.

38. Ibid.

39. Melissa A. Rosenfeld et al., "Adenovirus-Mediated Transfer of a Recombinant Alpha 1-Antitrypsin Gene to the Lung Epithelium in Vivo," *Science* 252(5004): 431–434; 19 April 1991; Richard C. Hubbard et al., "Anti-Neutrophil-Elastase Defenses of the Lower Respiratory Tract in Alpha 1-Antitrypsin Deficiency Directly Augmented with an Aerosol of Alpha 1-Antitrypsin," *Annals of Internal Medicine* 111(3): 206–212; 1 August 1989; Ronald G. Crystal et al., "The Alpha 1–Antitrypsin Gene and Its Mutations: Clinical Consequences and Strategies for Therapy," *Chest* 95(1): 196–208; January 1989.

40. Hubbard et al., op. cit.; Crystal et al., "The Alpha 1-Antitrypsin Gene."

41. Rosenfeld et al., op. cit.; Carol Ezzell, "Genetic Therapy: Just a Nasal Spray Away?" *Science News* 139(16): 246; 20 April 1991; Ronald Kotulak, "Technique May Fight Emphysema," *Chicago Tribune*, April 19, 1991, Section 1, p. 4; Andrew Skolnick, "Gene Replacement Therapy for Hereditary Emphysema?" *JAMA* 262(18): 2499; 10 November 1989; and Barbara J. Culliton, "Endothelial Cells to the Rescue," *Science* 246(4931): 750; 10 November 1989.

42. King and Stansfield, op. cit., p. 82; Theodore Friedmann, *Gene Therapy: Fact and Fiction in Biology's New Approaches to Disease* (Cold Spring Harbor, NY: Banbury Center, Cold Spring Harbor Laboratory, 1993), p. 126; Ezzell, "Genetic Therapy."

43. Ezzell, "Genetic Therapy" Beverly Merz, "Gene Therapy Enters 'Second Generation,'" *American Medical News*, December 22/29, 1989, pp. 3, 11.

44. P.L. Felgner and G. Rhodes, "Gene Therapeutics," *Nature* 349(6307): 351–352; 24 January 1991.

45. Ezzell, "Genetic Therapy."

46. Joseph Zabner et al., "Adenovirus-Mediated Gene Transfer Transiently Corrects the Chloride Transport Defect in Nasal Epithelia of Patients with Cystic Fibrosis," *Cell* 75(2): 207–216; 22 October 1993.

47. Ibid.

48. Ibid.

49. Kathy A. Fackelmann, "Glowing Evidence of Gene-Altered Arteries," *Science News* 139(25): 391; 22 June 1991.

50. Elizabeth G. Nabel et al., "Recombinant Gene Expression *in Vivo* Within Endothelial Cells of the Arterial Wall," *Science* 244(4910): 1342–1344; 16 June 1989. See also Culliton, op. cit. (note 41), p. 246.

51. Jerry E. Bishop, "Michigan Researchers Are Developing Method to Place Genes in Body Tissues," *Wall Street Journal*, September 14, 1990, p. B4; Elizabeth G. Nabel et al., "Site-Specific Gene Expression in Vivo by Direct Gene Transfer into the Arterial Wall," *Science* 249(4974): 1285–1288; 14 September 1990.

52. Nabel et al., "Site-Specific Gene Expression," p. 1287.

53. Culliton, op. cit. (note 41), p. 749. See also Leon Jaroff, "Giant Step for Gene Therapy," *Time*, September 24, 1990, pp. 74–76, chart on p. 76.

54. King and Stansfield, op. cit. (note 22), p. 46.

55. Brian E. Henderson et al., "Toward the Primary Prevention of Cancer," *Science* 254(5035): 1131–1138; 22 November 1991.

56. Ibid.

57. Natalie Angier, "New Gene Therapy to Fight Cancer Passes First Human Test," *New York Times*, July 18, 1991, p. B7; Carol Ezzell, "Scientists Seek to Fight Cancer with Cancer," *Science News* 139(21): 326; 25 March 1991; and Peter Gorner, "Panel OKs Gene Fight vs. Cancer," *Chicago Tribune*, August 1, 1990, Section 1, p. 5.

58. Paul T. Golumbek et al., "Treatment of Established Renal Cancer by Tumor Cells Engineered to Secrete Interleukin-4," *Science* 254(5032): 713–716; 1 November 1991; David Brown, "Cancer in Mice Is Cured by Gene Therapy, " *Washington Post*, November 1, 1991, p. A22.

59. Ezzell, "Scientists" Michael Waldholz, "Gene Implants Destroy Cancer In Lab Rodents," *Wall Street Journal*, November 1, 1991, p. B1.

Some of Rosenberg's peers suggested that this second round of cancer gene therapy experiments was premature and not grounded on solid scientific evidence. Drew Pardoll, whose research Rosenberg himself called "crucial to validating the human studies we are doing," stated that TNF was ineffective in catalyzing an enhanced immune response against cancer in animals (Waldholz, "Gene Implants"). However, even if this first attempt at stimulating patients' immune systems with gene therapy does not work, the idea remains promising and will probably be investigated using genes other than those for TNF.

60. Gary J. Nabel et al., "Immunotherapy of Malignancy by In Vivo Gene Transfer Into Tumors," Human Gene Therapy Protocol, submitted October 1991.

61. Robert A. Weinberg, "Tumor Suppressor Genes," *Science* 254(5035): 1138–1146; 22 November 1991.

62. Monica Hollstein et al., "p53 Mutations in Human Cancers," *Science* 253(5015): 49–53; 5 July 1991.

63. Weinberg, op. cit.

64. Ibid., p. 1145; Ruth Sager, "Tumor Suppressor Genes: The Puzzle and the Promise," *Science* 246(4936): 1406–1412; 15 December 1989.

65. Robert Bookstein et al., "Suppression of Tumorigenicity of Human Prostate Carcinoma Cells by Replacing a Mutated RB Gene," *Science* 247(4943): 712–715; 9 February 1990; and Beverly Merz, "Use of Anti-Oncogenes Studied," *American Medical News*, February 23, 1990, p. 8.

66. Arnold J. Levine et al., "The p53 Tumour Suppressor Gene," *Nature* 351(6326): 453–456; 6 June 1991; Weinberg, op. cit., p. 1143.

67. Hollstein et al., op. cit.

68. Levine et al., op. cit.; Weinberg et al., op. cit., p. 1143.

69. Weinberg, op. cit., p. 1143; Levine et al., op. cit., p. 454.

70. Suzanne J. Baker et al., "Suppression of Human Colorectal Carcinoma Cell Growth by Wild-Type p53," *Science* 249(4971): 912–915; 24 August 1990.

71. Michael Waldholz, "Colon Cancer Growth Is Halted in Tests By Replacing 'Tumor Suppressor' Genes," *Wall Street Journal*, August 24, 1990, p. B2.

72. Edward H. Oldfield et al., "Gene Therapy for the Treatment of Brain Tumors Using Intra Tumoral Transduction with the Thymidine Kinase Gene and Intravenous Ganciclovir," *Human Gene Therapy* 4(1): 39–69; February 1993.

73. Protocols 9306–044, 9306–054, 9306–054, 9406–077, as listed in the June 1995 Data Management Report, Office of Recombinant DNA Activities, National Institutes of Health.

74. Protocols 9409–084 (Holt/Arteaga) and 9306–052 (Ilan), abstracts.

75. Protocol 9306–048 (Galpin/Casciato), non-technical and scientific abstracts (1993).

76. Philip Greenberg et al., "A Phase I/II Study of Cellular Adoptive Immunotherapy Using Genetically Modified CD8+ HIV-Specific T Cells for HIV-Seropositive Patients Undergoing Allogeneic Bone Marrow Transplant," Human Gene Therapy Protocol, submitted October 1991.

77. W. French Anderson, "Gene Therapy for AIDS," *Human Gene Therapy* 5(2): 149–150; February 1994.

78. John Carey, "Gene Therapy: Cells That Carry Messengers of Health," *Business Week*, May 28, 1990, p. 74; Leon Jaroff, "Giant Step for Gene Therapy," *Time*, September 24, 1990, p. 76.

79. Anderson, "Gene Therapy for AIDS."

80. Ibid.

81. Friedmann, *Gene Therapy: Fact and Fiction*, (note 42), pp. 131–132; King and Stansfield, op. cit. (note 22), pp. 143, 291, 312.

82. Anderson, "Prospects for Human Gene Therapy," (note 8), p. 401.

83. King and Stansfield, op. cit. (note 22), p. 143.

84. Theodore Friedmann, "Progress Toward Human Gene Therapy," *Science* 244 (4910): 1275; 16 June 1989; David Suzuki and Peter Knudtson, *Genethics: The Clash Between the New Genetics and Human Values* (Cambridge, MA: Harvard University Press, 1989), p. 175.

85. Philippe Leboulch et al., "Mutagenesis of Retroviral Vectors Transducing Human Beta-Globin Gene and Beta-Globin Locus Control Region Derivatives Results in Stable Transmission of an Active Transcriptional Structure," *EMBO Journal* 13(13): 3065–3076; 1 July 1994.

86. Gina Kolata, "First Effort to Treat Muscular Dystrophy," *New York Times*, May 2, 1991, p. B10; Peter Gorner, "Gene Injections to Fight Muscular Dystrophy," *Chicago Tribune*, April 26, 1991, Section 1, p. 1; Felgner and Rhodes, op. cit. (note 44); Gina Kolata, "Why Gene Therapy Is Considered Scary But Cell Therapy Isn't," *New York Times*, September 16, 1990, p. E5. See also S.B. England et al., "Very Mild Muscular Dystrophy Associated with the Deletion of 46% of Dystrophin," *Nature* 343(6254): 180–182; 11 January 1990.

87. England, et al., p. 180.

88. Dr. Law has encountered resistance from some parts of the medical community, who believe his human experiments are premature. He has therefore severed his relationship with the Muscular Dystrophy Association and with the University of Tennessee and has established his own research entity, the Cell Therapy Research Foundation, within which he conducts his experiments after institutional review board (IRB) review.

89. Kolata, "First Effort."

90. See, for example, Arthur L. Caplan, H. Tristram Engelhardt, Jr., and James J. McCartney, eds., *Concepts of Health and Disease: Interdisciplinary Perspectives* (Reading, MA: Addison-Wesley, 1981); and H. Tristram Engelhardt, Jr., and Kevin Wm. Wildes, "Health and Disease. IV. Philosophical Perspectives," in Warren T. Reich, ed.-in-chief, *Encyclopedia of Bioethics* (revised ed.; New York: Simon and Schuster Macmillan, 1995), Vol. II, pp. 1101–1106.

91. Norman Daniels, *Just Health Care* (Cambridge: Cambridge University Press, 1985), esp. pp. 26–32; Christopher Boorse, "Health as a Theoretical Concept," *Philosophy of Science* 44(4): 542–573; December 1977; and Christopher Boorse, "On the Distinction Between Disease and Illness," *Philosophy and Public Affairs* 5(1): 49–68; Fall 1975.

92. Two helpful discussions of the just allocation of human gene therapy are Norman Daniels, "The Genome Project, Individuals, and Just Health Care," in Timothy F. Murphy and Marc A. Lappé, eds., *Justice and the Human Genome Project* (Berkeley: University of California Press, 1994), pp. 110–132; and Leonard M. Fleck, "Just Genetics: A Problem Agenda," pp. 133–152.

93. For discussion of this case, see Larry Thompson, "Healy Approves an Unproven Treatment," *Science* 259(5092): 172; 8 January 1993; and Larry Thompson, "Should Dying Patients Receive Untested Genetic Methods?," *Science* 259(5094): 452; 22 January 1993.

94. See, for example, Jay Katz, with Alexander Morgan Capron and Eleanor Swift Glass, *Experimentation with Human Beings: The Authority of the Investigator, Subject, Professions, and State in the Human Experimentation Process* (New York: Russell Sage Foundation, 1972).

95. See, for example, Anna C. Mastroianni, Ruth Faden, and Daniel Federman, eds., *Women and Health Research: Ethical and Legal Issues of Including Women in Clinical Studies* (2 vols.; Washington, DC: National Academy Press, 1994).

96. Larry Thompson, "The First Kids with New Genes," *Time*, June 7, 1993, pp. 50–53.

97. Leon Jaroff, "Brave New Babies," *Time*, May 31, 1993, pp. 56–57.

98. Gina Kolata, "Novel Bypass Method: A Dose of New Genes," *New York Times*, December 13, 1994, p. C1.

99. U.S., Congress, Office of Technology Assessment (OTA), *New Developments in Biotechnology—Background Paper: Public Perceptions of Biotechnology* (Washington, DC: U.S. Government Printing Office, May 1987).

100. March of Dimes (MOD) Birth Defects Foundation, "Genetic Testing and Gene Therapy Survey: Questionnaire and Responses" (White Plains, NY: March of Dimes Birth Defects Foundation, September 1992).

101. OTA, op. cit., p. 46, Table 28.

102. MOD, op. cit., p. 1, Question A1b.

103. OTA, op. cit., p. 71.

104. MOD, op. cit., p. 3. The heading for the table is the authors'.

105. OTA, p. 76, Table 58; MOD, p. 4. The heading is the authors'.

106. OTA, p. 77, Table 59; MOD, p. 4. The heading is the authors'.

107. OTA, p. 84, Table 63, Question (Q34).

108. MOD, Question A4, p. 2.

109. On common-morality theories, see Tom L. Beauchamp and James F. Childress, *Principles of Biomedical Ethics* (4th ed.; New York; Oxford University Press, 1994), pp. 100–111.

110. Darryl Macer, "Japanese Attitudes to Genetic Technology: National and International Comparisons," in Norio Fujiki and Darryl R.J. Macer, eds., *Human Genome Research and Society* (Christchurch, New Zealand: Eubios Ethics Institute, 1992), pp. 120–137.

111. See, for example, LeRoy Walters, "Ethics and New Reproductive Technologies: An International Review of Committee Statements," *Hastings Center Report* 17(3, Supplement): S3–S9; June 1987.

112. For a traditional defense of the role of wise people in guiding ethical judgments, see Thomas Aquinas, *Summa Theologiae*, I-II, question 95, 1 and 2.

113. For early discussion see Michael Hamilton, ed., *The New Genetics and the Future of Man* (Grand Rapids, MI: Eerdmans, 1972).

114. Eliot Marshall, "Gene Therapy's Growing Pains," *Science* 269(5227): 1050–1055; 25 August 1995. See also Gina Kolata, "In the Rush Toward Gene Therapy, Some See a High Risk of Failure," *New York Times*, July 25, 1995, p. C3.

115. For further discussion of this point, see Institute of Medicine, Division of Health Promotion and Disease Prevention, *New Vaccine Development: Establishing Priorities*, Volume I: *Diseases of Importance in the United States* (Washington, DC: National Academy Press, 1985), chapters 3 and 4.

116. For a summary of studies being conducted in countries other than the United States see a current issue of *Human Gene Therapy*. For a recent report on gene therapy research in the United Kingdom, see United Kingdom, Health Departments, Gene Therapy Advisory Committee, *First Annual Report: November 1993–December 1994* (London: Department of Health, January 1995).

117. Daniel Glick, "A Genetic Road Map," *Newsweek*, October 2, 1989, p. 46.

118. Ibid.

3

Germ-Line
Gene Therapy

Scientific Issues

Germ-Line Gene Therapy for Shiverer Mice

Though not yet attempted in humans, germ-line gene-transfer techniques have been much practiced in mice. The potential power of germ-line gene therapy can be illustrated by the example of shiverer mice, which suffer from tremors, convulsions, and early death caused by the lack of a nervous system protein called *myelin basic protein* (*MBP*).

MBP is an important building block of a substance known as *myelin* that coats the surface of nerve cells. Myelin serves some of the same purposes for a nerve cell as a rubber sheath serves for an electrical wire. Thus, it keeps the electrical impulses inside the cell from escaping and facilitates the conduction of electricity from one end of the nerve cell to the other. Without myelin, nervous impulses are lost and the nervous system has difficulty delivering instructions from one location to another.

A shiverer mouse cannot produce functional myelin because of a deletion mutation in the MBP gene. That is, the MBP gene is missing a significant stretch of DNA essential for encoding a functional MBP protein. The resulting abnormal myelination of a shiverer mouse's central nervous system produces the "shivering" and other symptoms described above. Although the shivering phenotype is not precisely analogous to a specific human disease, it does share some properties with multiple sclerosis, a disease of the human nervous system characterized by patches of dismyelination and corollary symptoms such as numbness, weakness, and impaired coordination.[1] Recent research has suggested that certain genes may increase a person's susceptibility to multiple sclerosis, which may be caused by an infectious agent.[2]

A group of researchers led by Leroy Hood of the California Institute of Technology has demonstrated that genetic alterations in the germ lines of shiverer mice can eliminate their symptoms. Hood and his colleagues first isolated and multiplied a segment of DNA that contained the MBP gene as well as some flanking sequences they suspected would be useful for correct expression of the gene. Then they microinjected approximately 200 copies of the DNA segment into each of 470 mouse *zygotes* (fertilized eggs).[3] Lastly, they reimplanted the zygotes in hormonally prepared foster mothers for gestation.[4]

From all of the injected and reimplanted zygotes, two mice were born that actually contained the added DNA segment (the *transgene*) in their cells. One of these two *transgenic* mice showed expression of the MBP gene.[5] This expressing transgenic mouse not only contained the transgene in her somatic cells; she also contained the transgene in her germ cells. The Hood team mated her with other mice and found that her transgene was passed on to her offspring. By crossbreeding the transgenic mouse with shiverer mice, the Hood team discovered that shiverer mice that inherited two copies of the transgene, in addition to their own partially deleted MBP genes, did not shiver. (On the other hand, shiverer mice that inherited only one copy of the transgene continued to exhibit shivering symptoms, suggesting that one copy of the properly functioning MBP allele cannot produce enough MBP to correct the shivering phenotype.) The MBP transgene in all of the transgenic mice was expressed in its normal tissue-specific manner and according to the proper developmental timing.[6] Thus, Hood and his colleagues successfully prevented tremors in shiverer mice and gave them normal life-spans by inserting the normal MBP gene into the germ lines of their parents.[7]

Besides Hood's group, several other research groups have prevented debilitating and life-threatening diseases in mice by genetically altering their germ lines.[8] In fact, there have been more demonstrated "cures" of laboratory animals through germ-line genetic intervention than through somatic cell gene therapy.

Potential Gene Therapy through Modification of Sperm Stem Cells

In November 1994 Ralph Brinster and his colleagues at the University of Pennsylvania announced a new method for transplanting sperm stem cells from one male mouse to another. If this new method were combined with techniques (as yet undeveloped) for genetically modifying sperm stem cells before transplantation, it would be possible to achieve germ-line gene therapy through modification of sperm stem cells. These cells are "the only self-renewing cell type in the adult capable of providing a genetic contribution to the next generation."[9] Brinster and his colleagues harvested sperm stem cells from donor mice, maintained the cells in vitro for several hours, and then transferred them into recipient male mice. The recipient mice were sterile, either because of a sterility-causing mutation or because they had been treated chemically to suppress their sperm cell production. The researchers were able to establish normal spermatogenesis in the previously-sterile recipient mice. In addition, the recipient mice produced mature spermatozoa that yielded offspring identifiable as derived from the donor sperm stem cells.

The researchers specifically express doubt that their technique can be used with mammalian egg cells because females possess the full complement of egg cells at birth; that is, no new egg cells are produced during the postnatal life of the female.[10] Nevertheless, Brinster and his colleagues have devised a procedure that holds promise for the treatment of male infertility and that ultimately may facilitate the development of methods for achieving germ-line gene transfer into gametes.[11]

Potential Advantages of Germ-Line Gene Therapy over Somatic Cell Therapy

Germ-line gene therapy involves a therapeutic genetic alteration in germ-line cells. As described in Chapter 1, the *germ line* includes gametes (reproductive cells, such as sperm and egg cells) as well as the cells from which they are derived. Germ-line gene therapy theoretically could be performed in sperm or egg cells, as in the Brinster et al. experiments described above. However, the vast majority of laboratory studies on germ-line approaches deal with the postfertilization stage, that is, with zygotes or preimplantation embryos.

A distinction should be drawn between germ-line effects that are unintended side effects of somatic cell gene therapy and interventions that are directly intended to have germ-line effects.[12] At the same time, however, we should note that there can be more than one intended target, or beneficiary, of germ-line gene therapy. In many cases, as in the case of the shiverer mice, germ-line gene therapy will be intended to serve the dual purposes of treating an individual (embryonic) "patient's" somatic cells *and* correcting a defect in that person's germ line.

In theory at least, germ-line gene therapy presents several advantages over somatic cell gene therapy. A gene that is added to a zygote (or to the cells of a preimplantation embryo) is passed down to daughter cells during cell division, along with the host zygote's genes. As a zygote develops into an embryo, a fetus, and then a child, all of its differentiating cells inherit the added gene, including somatic and germ cells. This result promises a clear benefit for the treatment of genetic diseases, such as cystic fibrosis, which affect many different organs and their disparate cell types.[13] Germ-line gene therapy would allow the addition of a properly functioning gene to all of the affected cell types in one fell swoop, whereas a combination of several separate somatic gene therapy procedures would likely be required to accomplish delivery to the same variety of cell types.

Germ-line gene therapy also presents an alternative to in vivo somatic cell gene therapy for diseases expressed in nonremovable cells and for diseases expressed in nondividing cells, which are intractable to many common somatic-cell gene-therapy techniques. (Lesch-Nyhan syndrome is an example of a disease expressed in the cells of the nervous system, which are both nonremovable and nondividing.)

In addition, because germ-line gene therapy would be performed at the earliest stages of human development, it presents the potential for preventing damage during fetal development that is attributable to defective genes. Somatic-cell gene therapy, which is by definition intended for differentiated cells, could not alleviate symptoms caused by irreversible damage that occurs during cell differentiation.[14]

Of course, in service of the goal of preventing genetic defects in the descendants of a patient, germ-line gene therapy would be superior to somatic cell gene therapy. For example, if a patient who suffers from sickle cell anemia wishes to prevent the disease in his children as well as to decrease the likelihood that his next-generation descendants will inherit the disease, a logical treatment choice would be germ-line gene therapy. Somatic gene therapy does not offer the potential to treat patients in such a comprehensive manner.

More broadly, germ-line gene therapy presents the prospect of reducing the incidence of certain inherited diseases in the human gene pool, whereas somatic cell gene therapy does not. That is, over a long period of time germ-line gene therapy could be used to decrease the frequency of malfunctioning genes—for example, the mutations that cause cystic fibrosis—and increase the frequency of properly functioning genes. Of course, such an improvement of the human gene pool could not be accomplished by merely treating individuals who suffer from genetic diseases. The great majority of defective genes reside in heterozygous individuals (those who have only one copy of a defective gene) who display normal phenotypes but can pass their disease-causing genes to future generations. In order to decrease the number of defective genes in the human gene pool, these phenotypically healthy *carriers* would have to be treated with germ-line gene therapy as well. An attempt to screen and treat heterozygotes who carry defective alleles is not an entirely unrealistic prospect. Programs of a similar scale have been carried out in order to counteract infectious diseases such as tuberculosis and smallpox.[15] Later in this chapter we will examine some of the ethical dimensions of such an ambitious public-health program.

Technical Matters

The potential methods for achieving human germ-line gene therapy vary depending upon the developmental stage at which gene transfer is envisioned. The technical steps for achieving germ-line gene therapy present a host of challenges. This section will present the developmental stages at which germ-line gene therapy might be achieved, potential methods, and the technical challenges that must be overcome before germ-line gene therapy will be reality. As will be explained, the overriding obstacle to germ-line gene therapy is our current inability to specify the site at which the needed gene integrates into the patients' cells.

Developmental stages at which germ-line gene transfer may be accomplished. Genes might be introduced into the human germ line at several different stages of human development. In the shiverer-mouse example given above, functioning genes were introduced into mouse zygotes, which are the single-celled precursors (that is, the fertilized eggs) from which all of the cells in an organism's body descend. Despite the differences between mice and humans, their developmental similarities suggest that the same genetic results would obtain in humans. Thus, if an introduced gene integrated into the genome of a human zygote, the resulting embryo should contain the added gene in all of its cells, including its germ cells.

What if an introduced gene integrated into one of the two cells of a two-cell human preimplantation embryo? Then the resulting later embryo would contain the added gene in half of its cells. Similarly, a gene that integrated into one of the four cells of a four-celled embryo should end up in one-fourth of the resulting embryo's cells, and so on.

At these very early stages of human development, cells have divided but not yet differentiated. Each cell still has the potential to differentiate into all of the different types of human cells that make up an adult human body. These early cells are therefore known as *totipotent* cells: They have total potential—the capacity to differentiate into all of the cells of the adult organism. As an embryo develops, and its cells begin to differentiate, these cells progressively lose their totipotency.[16] As long as cells retain their totipotency, genes added to them may end up in the germ line of the resulting person, as well as in every other type of human cell.

Another possible method of germ-line genetic alteration involves delivering genes directly into germ cells themselves—a possible extrapolation from the experiment on sperm stem cells in mice performed by Brinster and his colleagues.[17] Even though germ cells are themselves resident among the fully differentiated cells of an adult person, they each have the distinctive capacity to combine with another germ cell to form a totipotential cell. Delivering genes directly to germ cells would therefore also result in delivery to the totipotential cells that are formed when the germ cells combine with others, and therefore to all the cells of the daughter. Despite the striking success of Brinster's studies, the technical obstacles to precise genetic modification of sperm and egg cells remain formidable.

Techniques for performing germ-line gene therapy. The animal experiments discussed above and the human somatic-cell gene-therapy experiments discussed in Chapter 2 suggest that germ-line gene therapy in humans would necessitate the following steps. First, researchers must isolate and multiply copies of the essential gene. This step involves the same well-established recombinant DNA techniques used to isolate and multiply copies of genes for somatic cell gene therapy.

Second, assuming that human gene transfer will be performed in vitro, as it has been in all of the animal research to date, ova will need to be retrieved from a woman and sperm (or sperm stem cells) from a man. If genes are to be transferred into sperm or egg cells, the transfer will occur before fertilization. If the genes are to be transferred into zygotes or preimplantation embryos, the transfer will occur during or after in vitro fertilization. Thus, in principle at least, genes might be transferred into gametes, zygotes, or preimplantation embryos (Figure 3–1).

The option of transferring genes into healthy zygotes, and then crossbreeding to introduce functioning genes into defective germ lines, is not available in humans as it is in transgenic animals. Thus, the third step for human germ-line

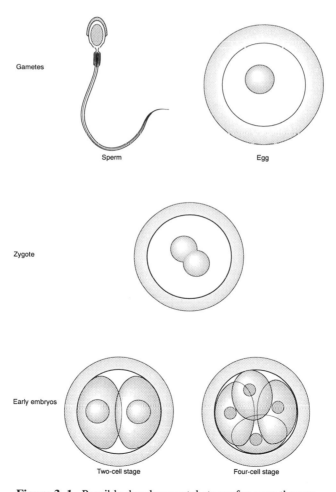

Figure 3–1. Possible developmental stages for gene therapy.

gene therapy must be to *detect* a mutation in a gamete, zygote, or preimplantation embryo, before it is expressed as a phenotype. This step represents a challenge that is particular to germ-line gene therapy and not present for somatic cell gene therapy. Before somatic cell gene therapy is performed, diseases can be diagnosed based upon patients' symptoms or genetic analysis of tissue samples (such as blood specimens). Germ-line gene therapy, on the other hand, requires that a genetic defect be diagnosed before the "patient" develops symptoms or even tissues. The germ-line gene therapy "patient" will be, at most, a zygote or preimplantation embryo at the time of gene transfer. (We do not regard sperm and egg cells as patients in any sense of that term.) Thus, diagnostic procedures that can be performed, in conjunction with in vitro fertilization, on gametes, preimplantation zygotes, or early embryos, are a prerequisite for germ-line gene therapy.

In fact, several clever *preimplantation diagnosis* techniques have been developed. The most important of these techniques involves the removal from an early (four- to eight-cell) embryo of one or two of its totipotential cells. The sample of DNA present in one or two totipotential cells is not large enough to analyze directly with currently available methods, but segments of the DNA can be analyzed by replicating them many times over (which is called *DNA amplification*).[18]

The growth of preimplantation diagnosis has been fueled by the 1983 invention of a technique called *polymerase chain reaction (PCR)*. PCR is a procedure that enables researchers to amplify DNA sequences with minimal time and energy. In addition to promising a revolutionary leap forward in preimplantation diagnostic capabilities, PCR has already promoted the flowering of an entire industry devoted to developing diagnostic tests for genetic diseases.[19] A parallel scientific development that also promises to foster preimplantation diagnosis advances is the Human Genome Project. By promoting the identification of genes associated with many new diseases, the Human Genome Project will undoubtedly accelerate the progress of preimplantation diagnostic procedures.

The fourth and most difficult step in germ-line gene therapy involves delivering functioning genes to gametes or totipotential cells. In connection with transgenic animal experiments and somatic cell gene transfer, several techniques have been developed for delivering genes into animal zygotes, preimplantation embryos, and separated totipotential cells. These in vitro techniques include virus-mediated delivery into early embryos,[20] microinjection into zygotes,[21] introduction of recombinant retroviruses into separated totipotent cells in culture,[22] transfection of totipotent cells in culture,[23] and homologous recombination into totipotent cells in culture.[24] Many of these techniques are similar to the techniques described in Chapter 2 for transferring genes into somatic cells. None of these methods has yet been tried in human zygotes, early embryos, or totipotential cells. However, theoretically, human germ-line gene therapy would entail applying these animal-tested methods to equivalent human cells.

Introducing genes directly into reproductive cells (gametes) themselves, a theoretically appealing method of delivering genes to the germ line, has not met with much success in animals. A strategy for transferring genes into sperm simply by mixing sperm with DNA in solution was reported successful in June 1989 by Italian researcher Corrado Spadafora. Although originally Spadafora's reports were greeted with great fanfare, eight other research teams that tried to duplicate his results reported that the experiment did not work.[25] However, the studies of mouse sperm stem cells by Brinster and his colleagues in November 1994 have given new impetus to this approach.[26]

Integration. After genes are transferred into the appropriate target cells, they generally integrate into the host genome. Integration is important for both successful gene expression and inheritance.[27] The site at which an added gene integrates into the host genome is even more significant to germ-line gene therapy than to somatic cell gene therapy. The site of integration bears on the efficiency of gene expression, the stability of the genetic alteration, and the risk of insertional mutation.

Introducing genes into gametes or totipotential cells does not automatically result in stable germ-line alteration. In order to reach viable germ lines, added genes must integrate into germ cells, zygotes, or preimplantation embryos without disrupting the development of the resulting fetuses. Perhaps the most significant technical obstacle to human germ-line gene transfer is our present inability to specify the site at which an added gene integrates, which may affect both development and heredity. Nonspecific integration is a technical obstacle for somatic cell gene therapy, too, but it presents a more significant problem for germ-line gene transfer for several reasons. First, an added gene may integrate into a zygote or embryo's genome at an inappropriate location and thereby create a dominant condition that is lethal to the developing individual, resulting in the death of the whole organism. By contrast, such a mutation in a particular somatic cell may only result in the death of that cell. (It is also possible, however, that an integrational mutation may result in a cancer that will ultimately lead to the death of a germ-line or somatic-cell gene-therapy patient.)

Second, a gene may integrate into a zygote's or embryo's genome at an inappropriate location and thereby create a mutation in one copy of any of an individual's essential genes. An insertional mutation in an essential gene, in a zygote or embryo, may result in the development of a heterozygous lethal mutation, transferable to the treated individual's offspring. By contrast, the consequences of an insertional mutation in an essential gene of a particular somatic cell may be trivial.

Third, if an added gene creates an insertional mutation in a zygote or embryo which is not incompatible with life but which threatens the health of the resulting individual, that insertional mutation has the potential to harm future generations as well as the current patient. Similar insertional mutations in somatic cells affect only the treated patient.

Fourth, even if undirected integration does not produce an insertional mutation in the host genome, it is inadequate for germ-line gene therapy because it does not stably correct the germ line. The benefits conferred by the addition of a functioning gene that integrates at a locus removed from its defective counterpart will often be lost during meiotic cell division, when the transgene can segregate away from its defective counterpart (Figure 3-2A and B). That is, during the meiotic

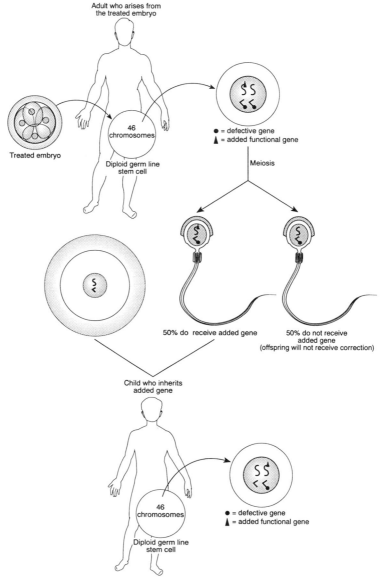

Figure 3–2A. Germ-line addition therapy: losing added gene during meiosis.

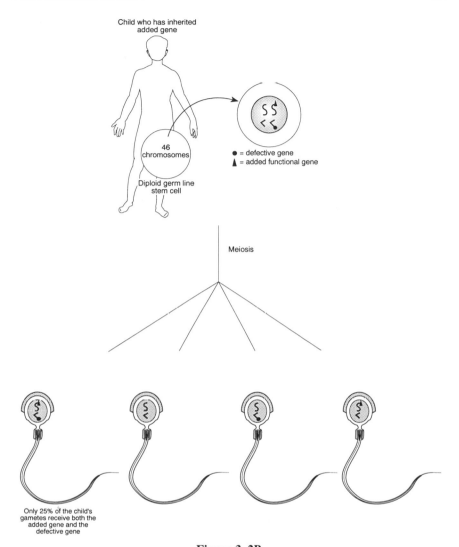

Child who has inherited
added gene

46
chromosomes

● = defective gene
▲ = added functional gene

Diploid germ line
stem cell

Meiosis

Only 25% of the child's
gametes receive both the
added gene and the
defective gene

Figure 3–2B.

cell division that reduces a diploid cell to haploid cells, the transgene and the defective allele may be parsed into separate gametes. As a result, some individuals
of the next generation will not receive the benefit of the genetic correction, even
though it has reached the parent's germ line.

Expression. Moreover, another hurdle stands in the way of germ-line gene
therapy. Even if the transgene is integrated in every cell in a person's body, germ-
line gene therapy will not be successful unless the transgene is properly expressed.
Factors that may impact gene expression include the site of integration, the com-
pleteness of the introduced DNA sequence, and chemical changes in the introduced DNA.

Gene expression, like gene integration, must be even more precise in connection with germ-line gene therapy than with somatic cell gene therapy. Like genes added to cells for somatic cell gene therapy, germ-line transgenes affect the somatic cells of the adult individuals in which they reside. In addition, however, transgenes affect fetal development and heredity. Therefore, the time and place in which transgenes are expressed have significant additional consequences in connection with germ-line gene therapy. The level of precision required for successful somatic cell gene therapy is insufficient for successful germ-line gene therapy. Germ-line gene therapy will not be ready to proceed until researchers are able to regulate more precisely gene expression in human cells.

In fact, unless a gene is properly expressed, a genetic alteration intended to correct an individual's germ line may never be transferred to the next generation. Many severe genetic diseases interfere with reproductive abilities or result in death before reproductive age. Patients suffering from such diseases will not be able to transmit genetic corrections through their germ lines unless the transgene corrects the deficiencies in their own bodies, enabling those patients to live to reproductive age and to regain their reproductive capacities.

Chimeras. Some (but not all) of the currently existing germ-line gene transfer methods, when used to transfer genes into cells of early mice embryos, generate a phenomenon called a *chimera*. A chimera (the word comes from the Greek mythological character who had a lion's head, a goat's body, and a serpent's tail[28]) is an individual composed of a mixture, or *mosaic*, of cells that are genetically different.[29] Germ-line gene transfer techniques involving totipotent cells in culture produce chimeras because they bestow genetic alterations only upon a portion of the cells of the resulting embryos. In these experiments, cultured, genetically altered totipotent cells are added to early embryos (in the blastocyst or morula stage) after several cell divisions and some differentiation of the host cells have already occurred. Only cells descended from the cultured totipotent cells contain the genetic alteration (Figure 3-3). Thus, gene transfer chimeras have transgenes in only a fraction of their germ-line cells, that is, only those germ-line cells descended from the embryonic cells that received the gene.

Even microinjection into a single-celled zygote does not insure against chimeras. An introduced gene's rate of integration into the host cell genome may limit the percentage of descendant cells that inherit that transgene. If an introduced gene integrates during the one-cell stage, all of the person's cells will inherit it. However, a gene that is microinjected at the one-cell stage might not integrate until the two-cell stage, when it will change the genome of only one of the two cells. Then only half of the embryo's cells will inherit the added gene and the resulting person will be a chimera. On the other hand, this delayed integration occurs only rarely in animal microinjection experiments and is therefore likely to be rare in microinjected human zygotes.[30]

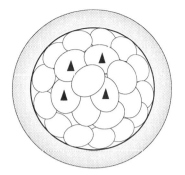

Genetically altered totipotential cells added to early embryos

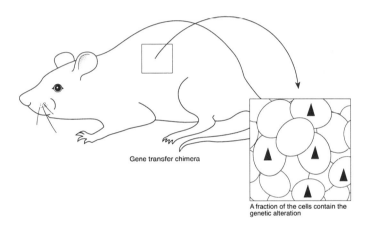

Gene transfer chimera

A fraction of the cells contain the
genetic alteration

Figure 3–3. Chimera.

In mice, chimeras can be bred to produce progeny that contain the genetic alteration in all of their cells. The progeny that result from the germ cells containing the added gene will have that gene in all of their cells. In humans, however,
using breeding as a method to produce individuals who contain genetic alterations
in all of their cells is impractical and raises troubling questions. Thus, in humans,
gene transfer into human germ cells could not be dependably accomplished via
chimeras. Nevertheless, certain genetic diseases may be effectively treated by
genetic correction of fewer than all of a patient's cells. (For example, somatic gene
therapy of ADA deficiency has been successful despite the fact that only a portion of each patients' cells have been genetically altered.) Thus, chimeric germ-
line gene therapy presents a potential option for the somatic treatment of some

genetic diseases in individual patients.[31] In addition, although chimeric alteration does not ensure that all of a patient's germ-line cells receive a genetic correction, it at least improves that "odds" that some of a patient's germ-line cells (and therefore, some of the patient's descendants) will receive the correction.

The Needed Technical Breakthrough: Gene Replacement

An improvement in gene transfer technology that allowed molecular biologists to direct inserted genes to specific sites would logarithmically enhance gene therapy. The position where an introduced gene integrates on a host cell chromosome influences the regulation of its expression. Thus, the ability to specify an insertion site would give researchers better control over gene expression. This much-desired technological improvement would also allow researchers to steer introduced genes away from inappropriate loci, where they might cause harm by awakening slumbering oncogenes, disrupting tumor-suppressor genes, or otherwise disturbing cell function in a way that would be risky to a patient.

The developers of gene therapy hope ultimately for more than the ability to direct the insertion site of added genes; they want the even more powerful capacity to replace disease-causing genes with functioning versions. Whereas presently available gene therapy methods can be descriptively labeled *gene addition therapy*, the desired technique would be more appropriately called *gene replacement therapy* or *gene surgery*. In an ideal example of this coveted technique, a gene therapist would excise a defective gene and cleanly replace it with a functioning version.

The difference between gene addition and gene replacement can be illustrated by an analogy from word processing. Gene addition is similar to giving the *insert* command in a word processing program. Researchers ask a vector to insert a properly functioning gene (a correctly spelled word) somewhere—anywhere—in a cell (document). After the insertion in a random site the cell is likely to function better than it had before because of the dynamic capabilities of cells. (A document with a randomly inserted properly spelled word would be less likely to be considered *corrected*.) In contrast, gene replacement is analogous to the global search-and-replace function in word processing programs. In this case the vector looks for a particular incorrect combination of letters (or even *any* combination of letters between two correct known letters) and replaces the original combination with a properly functioning gene (correctly spelled word).

Clean and precise replacement would be advantageous in several ways. The added gene, residing in its normal locus, would be more likely to be appropriately regulated and expressed. Just as a plant in its normal habitat gets the correct amount of sunlight, moisture, and nutrients, a gene in its normal locus gets the right amount of transcription, splicing, and translation.

In addition, a gene inserted into its normal locus would be less likely to disturb cell function. Gene replacement would reduce or eliminate a significant risk presented by gene addition—that the added gene will disrupt an essential gene by inserting directly into one of its coding or regulatory sequences.

Gene replacement therapy would also be superior to gene addition therapy because of its potential to cure dominant as well as recessive diseases.[32] Certain dominant genetic diseases are caused by malfunctioning genes that are expressed at inappropriate times or in inappropriate cells. Gene addition therapy's introduction of a properly functioning version of the defective gene would not erase the presence of one of these unfit products.[33] On the other hand, gene replacement therapy could cure such dominant genetic diseases by eliminating the gene that produces the inappropriate product and replacing it with a normal gene that does not (Figure 3-4).

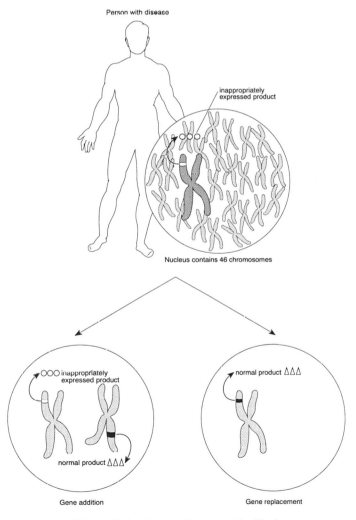

Person with disease

inappropriately
expressed product

Nucleus contains 46 chromosomes

OOO inappropriately
expressed product

normal product △△△

normal product △△△

Gene addition

Gene replacement

Figure 3–4. Gene replacement: the ideal.

Gene replacement has been achieved in cells in vitro using elegant and creative scientific strategies that take advantage of a naturally occurring phenomenon called *homologous recombination*.[34] (See Appendix E for technical details about homologous recombination.) Homologous recombination is a mechanism by which foreign DNA sequences integrate into host cell chromosomes at sites where the host DNA sequences are homologous (fundamentally similar). Harnessing homologous recombination for directed use in human cells would go a long way toward achieving gene replacement therapy. As a potential future refinement of current gene therapy techniques, gene replacement therapy mediated by homologous recombination is among the most promising.

The Potential Usefulness of Human Germ-Line Gene Therapy

If germ-line gene therapy becomes technically viable, will it be used? In answering this question, it should first be recognized that germ-line gene therapy serves the purpose of treating genetic disease either before or shortly after the conception of the "patient(s)" who will be treated. The utility of germ-line gene therapy depends, at least in part, on the availability and effectiveness of alternative medical procedures for the treatment and prevention of genetic disease. Although there are no other medical techniques for treating genetic diseases in patients at this very early stage in their life cycles, there are other medical techniques that can promise treatment at later stages in a patient's life. Standard medical treatment and somatic cell gene therapy administered to successive generations may present viable alternatives to germ-line gene therapy for some diseases. For example, it may ultimately become a technically simple matter to treat alpha 1-antitrypsin deficiency with somatic gene therapy administered via inhalation of viral vectors carrying a functional AAT gene. (See pp. 28–29 above.) The ability to provide uncomplicated and effective somatic cell gene therapy to successive generations of patients may then obviate the need to resort to germ-line gene therapy, which will probably be more risky and complicated.

Prenatal diagnosis followed by selective abortion and preimplantation diagnosis followed by selection of unaffected embryos present additional alternatives for the prevention of genetic disease in repeated generations. For prenatal diagnosis, fetal testing by chorionic villi sampling or amniocentesis can be used to determine the presence of a variety of genetic diseases, such as Tay-Sachs disease and cystic fibrosis. For preimplantation selection, zygotes or early embryos can be tested in vitro after fertilization; then only the genetically healthy embryos will be transferred. These alternatives are feasible because two parents who both carry recessive-disease-causing genes have a 75% chance of producing a healthy child (Figure 3-5). For nonrecessive diseases, that percentage may vary. Nevertheless, as long as some percentage of a couple's children are expected to be healthy, the option exists to diagnose the genetic defect at the embryonic stage or

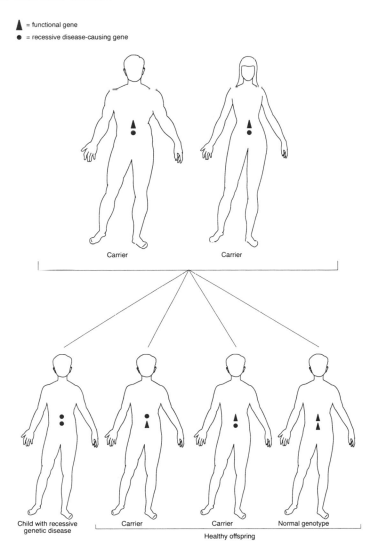

Figure 3–5. Possible genotypes of children of parents who both carry recessive disease-causing genes.

the fetal stage and then to allow the development only of the disease-free individuals to continue. Prenatal diagnosis followed by abortion is already a widely used method of preventing genetic disease. Preimplantation selection is an option offered at a growing number of fertility centers. Both of these alternatives may provide less risky and less expensive methods of preventing genetic disease than germ-line gene therapy. At the same time, however, it must be acknowledged that these strategies do not attempt to treat the affected embryos or fetuses.

One example of preimplantation diagnosis can be found in studies by British scientists who tested eight-cell human embryos by removing one of the cells and using PCR to analyze the genome. These tests were performed in order to determine the sex of embryos of couples at risk for producing male children who suffered from male-specific genetic diseases. (Such diseases, called X-linked diseases, are further described in Appendix B.) Subsequent to these preimplantation diagnoses, female embryos were transferred to the mothers for gestation, and with a reasonably high success rate, these embryos produced healthy female children.[35]

It should be recognized that the various alternatives for approaching genetic disease have differing effects on the germ line of the treated patient. Standard medical therapies, like somatic cell gene therapy, are somatic treatments and do not correct genetic defects in a patient's germ line. They may allow patients to live and to reproduce, passing on genetic mistakes which, without treatment, would not be perpetuated. Preimplantation and prenatal selection, like somatic medicine, may also result in a higher incidence of germ-line genetic defects because, unless they employ selective discard and selective abortion of unaffected carriers, both strategies increase the number of carriers of genetic defects that are born.

Successful germ-line gene replacement, on the other hand, will not perpetuate genetic mistakes. It will not only cure the patient at hand; it will also prevent the disease in question from arising in that patient's descendants. Applied to heterozygous carriers on a large scale, it could theoretically eliminate chosen disease-causing genes from the human gene pool.

As long as germ-line gene therapy must be performed on human zygotes or embryos one at a time after in vitro fertilization, it is likely to remain an expensive technology with limited use. Only if a technique is developed for performing gene replacement or gene repair within the reproductive cells of human adults—perhaps through the injection of highly refined vectors that "home in" only on those cells (or their precursors in males)—are we likely to see the widespread diffusion of germ line genetic intervention for disease prevention.

Ethical Issues

An Earlier Stage of the Discussion: Muller versus Lederberg

The ethical debate[36] over intentionally introducing genetic changes into the human germ line through advanced biomedical techniques goes back at least to the 1920s and 1930s and the writings of classical geneticists J.B.S. Haldane[37] and H.J. Muller.[38] The discussion was renewed in the late 1950s and early 1960s, with two of the chief protagonists being H.J. Muller and molecular biologist Joshua Lederberg. Muller advocated the improvement of the gene pool through voluntary programs of assisted reproduction—specifically artificial insemination using semen from donors who had what Muller viewed as the best combination of physical, intellectual, and moral qualities.[39] (Egg donation was not a technical possibility in the 1960s, as it is today. Given his general advocacy of women's rights, Muller would surely have approved the equal participation of women in this voluntary program for improving the human gene pool.) At a symposium held in London in November 1962, Joshua Lederberg criticized Muller's proposal for its lack of precision and for the very slow progress that Muller's plan for guided evolution would deliver. In Lederberg's words,

The recent achievements of molecular biology strengthen our eugenic means to achieve [human survival]. But do they necessarily support proposals to transfer animal husbandry to man? My own first conclusion is that the technology of human genetics is pitifully clumsy, even by the standards of practical agriculture. Surely within a few generations we can expect to learn tricks of immeasurable advantage. Why bother now with somatic selection, so slow in its impact? Investing a fraction of the effort, we should soon learn how to manipulate chromosome ploidy [number of sets of chromosomes], homozygosis [the union of gametes that are identical for one or more pairs of genes], gametic selection, full diagnosis of heterozygotes, to accomplish in one or two generations of eugenic practice what would now take ten or one hundred.[40]

Even 30+ years after Lederberg's statement there are many "tricks" that molecular biologists have not yet learned about genes, chromosomes, and cells. The chief trick that remains elusive is guiding new genes to precise locations where they can replace malfunctioning genes. Also, in the 1990s we are less likely to *begin* our discussions of germ-line genetic intervention by thinking of global effects on human evolution. We are much more likely to begin by considering specific diseases and decisions that are likely to be faced by couples who are deciding whether or not to have children. The thinking of those couples will be focused, first and foremost, on the welfare of their children and perhaps on the welfare of their children's children as well.

A Preliminary Question: Should This Issue Be Discussed at All?

In September of 1992 a distinguished physician–scientist, Dr. James V. Neel, appeared before the NIH RAC to discuss spontaneous and induced germ-line mutation. Dr. Neel argued that it would be premature for the RAC to discuss the scientific and ethical questions surrounding germ-line gene therapy. His precise message, as summarized in a 1993 editorial, was the following:

The Committee's desire to prepare itself for future developments would under most circumstances be laudable, but for a Committee with this visibility and prestige to begin to consider the subject of germ-line therapy in an organized fashion at this time would send the wrong vibes to the scientific, ethical, and political communities. Such an action might appear to imply the belief that the Committee would be seriously considering this prospect within the terms of office of present Committee members. Given the tremendous issues at stake, and even with the utmost attempt on my part to anticipate the amazing speed of advances in the field of molecular genetics, I could not imagine serious organized discussions of this subject by such a group within the next 20 or 30 years. (Individuals will, of course, express their views as they please.)[41]

Dr. Neel carefully avoids urging individuals, like the present authors, to refrain from discussing the topic of germ-line gene therapy. On the other hand, he clearly thinks that it would be a mistake for public advisory committees like the RAC to engage in anticipatory discussions of this subject. We respectfully disagree. In our view, the years from 1983 through 1988, during which the RAC looked ahead to the first hypothetical somatic-cell gene-therapy proposals, were very profitably devoted to anticipating what the new technology might mean and to developing "points to consider," or very general guidelines, for somatic cell therapy proposals. In a similar way, given the research advances outlined in the earlier part of this chapter, we think that both individuals and public advisory committees would be wise to begin the discussion of this important topic sooner rather than later. If proposals for human application of germ-line gene therapy are delayed because of technical obstacles, or if research moves in unanticipated directions that must then later be taken into account, the risks of premature discussion are low. On the other hand, if a technical breakthrough occurs that makes germ-line gene therapy feasible, the anticipatory discussion of the topic may turn out to have been essential for the calm formulation of rational oversight policies.

For What Clinical Situations Will Germ-Line Gene Therapy Be Proposed?

It is difficult to predict the precise context in which germ-line gene therapy will be first be considered. Tables 3-1 through 3-4 show four scenarios where the issue of germ-line intervention may at least be discussed at some point in the future.

The kind of situation described in Table 3-1 is likely to arise as medical care succeeds in prolonging the lives of people with genetic disorders such as sickle cell disease or cystic fibrosis. If somatic cell gene therapy is employed in significant numbers of people afflicted with recessive genetic diseases, some of those people's somatic cells will be able to function normally, but their reproductive cells will remain unchanged, thus assuring that they will be carriers of genetic disease to the next generation. If two such phenotypically cured people marry and

Table 3-1 Mode of Inheritance 1

Both the wife and the husband are afflicted with a recessive genetic disorder. That is, both have two copies of the same malfunctioning gene at a particular site in their chromosomes. Therefore, all of their offspring are likely to be affected with the same genetic disorder.

have children, all or almost all of their children will be afflicted with the disease which their parents had. Each succeeding generation of these children will need somatic cell gene therapy for the treatment of their disease.

Table 3-2 sketches a scenario frequently encountered by genetic counselors. In this case, germ-line genetic intervention could be viewed as an alternative to pre-natal diagnosis and selective abortion of affected fetuses or to preimplantation diagnosis and the selective discard of affected early embryos. A couple might also elect germ-line genetic intervention in order to avoid producing children who are *carriers* of genetic defects, even if the children are not themselves afflicted with genetic disease. The parents would know that children who are carriers may one day face precisely the kind of difficult reproductive decisions that they as parents are facing.

In the type of case outlined in Table 3-3, somatic cell gene therapy might be effective if one could deliver it to the developing embryo and fetus during the earliest stages of pregnancy, that is, shortly after the embryo has implanted in the uterus. However, there is no known method of administering intrauterine therapy to an early first-trimester embryo, and a deferral of treatment until the second or third trimester would probably allow irreversible damage to occur. Preimplanta-tion treatment, which would almost certainly affect the future germ-line cells as well as the future somatic cells, could be the only feasible approach to producing children who are not brain damaged, especially for couples who reject the alter-native of selectively discarding early embryos.[42]

The scenario presented in Table 3-4 may be especially relevant to the develop-ment of particular kinds of cancers as a result of inborn genetic factors and subse-quent mutations. For example, about 40% of people with a cancer of the retina called *retinoblastoma* transmit a dominant gene for this disorder to their children. In patients with this germ-line type of retinoblastoma, somatic mutational events that occur after birth seem to activate the cancer-causing gene and can result in multiple types of cancer developing in different cell types within the patient's body. For example, a kind of cancer called *osteogenic sarcoma* frequently develops later in life in patients who have been successfully treated for retinoblastoma.[43] With germ-line retinoblastoma, the only effective antidote to the development of mul-tiple types of cancers may be early germ-line gene therapy that effectively repairs *all* of the cells in a developing embryo.[44]

Table 3-2 Mode of Inheritance 2

Both the wife and the husband are carriers of a recessive genetic disorder. That is, each has one copy of a properly functioning and one copy of a malfunctioning gene at a particular site in their chromosomes. Following Mendel's laws, 25% of the couple's offspring are likely to be "normal," 50% are likely to be carriers like their parents, and 25% are likely to be afflicted with the genetic disorder.

Table 3-3 Disease Condition 1

A diagnosable genetic disorder results in major, irreversible damage to the brains of affected fetuses during the first trimester of pregnancy. There is no known method for making genetic repairs in the uterus during pregnancy. If any genetic repair is to be made, it must be completed before the embryo begins its intrauterine development.

Table 3-4 Disease Condition 2

A diagnosable genetic disorder affects many different cell types in many different parts of the bodies of patients affected by the disorder. Somatic cell gene therapy that targets a particular cell type is therefore unlikely to be successful in combating the disorder. Therefore, germ-line gene therapy delivered early enough to affect *all* cell types may be the only feasible way to prevent disease in a particular future person.

The Needed Technological Breakthrough: Gene Replacement or Gene Repair

As we noted earlier in this chapter, the current technique for somatic-cell gene therapy relies on rather imprecise methods of gene addition. For safe and effective germ-line gene therapy, it seems likely that a more precisely targeted method of gene replacement or gene repair will be necessary. The most obvious reason for preferring gene replacement is that gene addition in embryos would result in their (later-developing) sperm or egg cells containing *both* the malfunctioning and the properly functioning genes. Thus, one undesirable effect of researchers' treating present or future reproductive cells by gene addition is that the researchers would be directly contributing to an increase in the number of malfunctioning genes in future generations. In addition, if any of the germ-line disorders are dominant, as retinoblastoma seems to be, then only gene replacement is likely to eradicate the deleterious effects of the malfunctioning gene.

Major Ethical Arguments in Favor of Germ-Line Gene Therapy

In this and the following section we will analyze the major ethical arguments[45] for and against germ-line gene therapy.[46] For this analysis we will make the optimistic assumption that germ-line intervention methods will gradually be refined until they reach the point where gene replacement or gene repair is technically feasible and able to be accomplished in more than 95% of attempted gene transfer procedures. Thus, the following analysis presents the arguments for and against germ-line intervention under the most favorable conditions for such intervention.

A first argument in favor of germ-line intervention is that it may be the only way to prevent damage to particular biological individuals when that damage is caused by certain kinds of genetic defects. This argument is most closely related to the last two scenarios presented above. That is, only genetic modifications introduced into preimplantation embryos are likely to be early enough to affect all of the important cell types (as in retinoblastoma), or to reach a large enough fraction of brain cells, or to be in time to prevent irreversible damage to the developing embryo. In these circumstances the primary intent of gene therapy would, or at least could, be to provide gene therapy for the early embryo. A side effect of the intervention would be that all of the embryonic cells, including the reproductive cells that would later develop, would be genetically modified.[47]

A second moral argument for germ-line genetic intervention might be advanced by parents. It is that they wish to spare their children and grandchildren from either (1) having to undergo somatic cell gene therapy if they are born affected with a genetic defect or (2) having to face difficult decisions regarding possibly transmitting a disease-related gene to their own children and grandchildren. In our first scenario, admittedly a rare case, two homozygous parents who have a genetic disease know in advance that all of their offspring are likely to be affected with the same genetic disease. In the second scenario, there is a certain probability that the parents' offspring will be affected or carriers. An assumption lying behind this second argument is that parents should enjoy a realm of moral and legal protection when they are making good-faith decisions about the health of their children. Only if their decisions are clearly adverse to the health interests of the children should moral criticism or legal intervention be considered.

A third moral argument for germ-line intervention is more likely to be made by health professionals, public-health officials, and legislators casting a wary eye toward the expenditures for health care. This argument is that, from a social and economic point of view, germ-line intervention is more efficient than repeating somatic cell gene therapy generation after generation. From a medical and public health point of view, germ-line intervention fits better with the increasingly preferred model of disease prevention and health promotion. In the very long run, germ-line intervention, if applied to both affected individuals and asymptomatic carriers of serious genetic defects, could have a beneficial effect on the human gene pool and the frequency of genetic disease.[48]

A fourth argument refers to the roles of researchers and health professionals. As a general rule, researchers deserve to have the freedom to explore new modes of treating and/or preventing human disease.[49] To be sure, moral rules set limits on how this research is conducted. For example, animals involved in the preclinical stages of the research should be treated humanely. In addition, the human subjects involved in the clinical trials should be treated with respect. When and if germ-line gene therapy is some day validated as a safe and effective intervention, health care providers should be free to, and may have a moral obligation to, offer it to their patients as a possible treatment. This freedom is based on the professional's general obligation to seek out and offer the best possible therapeutic alternatives to patients and society's recognition of a sphere in which health professionals are at liberty to exercise their best judgment on behalf of their patients.

A fifth and final argument in favor of germ-line gene therapy is that this kind of intervention best accords with the health professions' healing role and with the concern to protect rather than penalize individuals who have disabilities. This argument is not simply a plea for protecting all embryos and fetuses from the time of fertilization forward. Both authors of this book think that abortion is morally justifiable in certain circumstances. However, prenatal diagnosis followed by selective abortion and preimplantation diagnosis followed by selective discard seem to us to be uncomfortable and probably discriminatory halfway technologies that should eventually be replaced by effective modes of treatment. The options of selective abortion and selective discard essentially say to prospective parents, "There is nothing effective that the health care system has to offer. You may want to give up on this fetus or embryo and try again." To people with disabilities that are diagnosable at the prenatal or preimplantation stages of development the message of selective abortion and selective discard may seem more threatening. That message may be read as, "If we health professionals and prospective parents had known you were coming, we would have terminated your development and attempted to find or create a nondisabled replacement."

This argument is not intended to limit the legal access of couples to selective abortion in the case of serious health problems for the fetus. We support such access. Rather, it is an argument about what the long-term goal of medicine and society should be. In our view, that long-term goal should be to prevent disability and disease wherever possible. Where prevention is not possible, the second-best alternative is a cure or other definitive remedy. In cases where neither prevention nor cure is possible, our goal should be to help people cope with disability and disease while simultaneously seeking to find a cure.

Major Arguments against Germ-Line Gene Therapy

First, if the technique has unanticipated negative effects, those effects will be visited not only on the recipient of the intervention himself or herself but also on all of the descendants of that recipient. This argument seems to assume that a mistake, once made, could not be corrected, or at least that the mistake might not become apparent until the recipient became the biological parent of at least one child. For that first child, at least, the negative effects could be serious, as well as uncorrectable.

Second, some critics of germ-line genetic intervention argue that this technique will never be necessary because of available alternative strategies for preventing the transmission of diagnosable genetic diseases. Specifically, critics of germ-line gene therapy have sometimes suggested that preimplantation diagnosis and the selective discard of affected embryos might be a reasonable alternative to the high-technology, potentially risky attempt to repair genetic defects in early human embryos. Even without in vitro fertilization and preimplantation diagnosis, the option of prenatal diagnosis and selective abortion is available for many disorders. According to this view, these two types of selection, before embryos or fetuses have reached the stage of viability, are effective means for achieving the same goal.

The third argument is closely related to the second: this technique will always be an expensive option that cannot be made available to most couples, certainly not by any publicly funded health care system. Therefore, like in vitro fertilization for couples attempting to overcome the problem of infertility, germ-line gene therapy will be available only to wealthy people who can afford to pay its considerable expense on their own.

The fourth argument builds on the preceding two: precisely because germ-line intervention will be of such limited utility in preventing disease, there will be strong pressures to use this technique for genetic enhancement at the embryonic stage, when it could reasonably be expected to make a difference in the future life prospects of the embryo. Again in this case, only the affluent would be able to afford the intervention. However, if enhancement interventions were safe and efficacious, the long-term effect of such germ-line intervention would probably be to exacerbate existing differences between the most-well-off and the least-well-off segments of society.

Fifth, even though germ-line genetic intervention aims in the long run to treat rather than to abort or discard, the issue of appropriate respect for preimplantation embryos and implanted fetuses will nonetheless arise in several ways. After thoroughgoing studies of germ-line intervention have been conducted in nonhuman embryos, there will undoubtedly be a stage at which parallel studies in human embryos will be proposed. The question of human embryo research was recently studied by a committee appointed by the director of the National Institutes of Health.[50] Although the committee specifically avoided commenting on germ-line intervention, its recommendation that certain kinds of human embryo research should be continued and that such research should be funded by NIH provoked considerable controversy. Critics of the committee's position would presumably also oppose the embryo research that would be proposed to prepare the way for germ-line gene therapy in humans.[51] Their principal argument would be that the destruction or other harming of preimplantation embryos in research is incompatible with the kind of respect that should be shown to human embryos.

Even after the research phase of germ-line genetic intervention is concluded, difficult questions about the treatment of embryos will remain. For example, preimplantation diagnosis may continue to involve the removal of one or two totipotential cells from a four- to eight-cell embryo. While the moral status of totipotential human embryonic cells has received scant attention in bioethical debates, there is at least a plausible argument that a totipotential cell, once separated from the remainder of a preimplantation embryo, is virtually equivalent to a zygote; that is, under favorable conditions it could develop into an embryo, a fetus, a newborn, and an adult. This objection to the destruction of totipotential embryonic cells will only be overcome if a noninvasive genetic diagnostic test for early embryos (like an x-ray or a CT scan) can be developed. Further, even if a noninvasive diagnostic test is available, as we have noted above, a postintervention diagnostic test will probably be undertaken with each embryo to verify that the intervention has been successful. Health professionals and prospective parents will probably be at least open to the possibility of selective discard or selective abortion if something has gone radically wrong in the intervention procedure. Thus, germ-line genetic intervention may remain foreclosed as a moral option to those who are conscientiously opposed to any action that would directly terminate the life of a preimplantation embryo or a fetus.

The sixth argument points to potential perils of concentrating great power in the hands of human beings. According to this view, the technique of germ-line intervention would give human beings, or a small group of human beings, too much control over the future evolution of the human race. This argument does not necessarily attribute malevolent intentions to those who have the training that would allow them to employ the technique. It implies that there are built-in limits that humans ought not to exceed, perhaps for theological or metaphysical reasons, and at least hints that corruptibility is an ever-present possibility for the very powerful.

The seventh argument explicitly raises the issue of malevolent use. If one extrapolates from Nazi racial hygiene programs, this argument asserts, it is likely the germ-line intervention will be used by unscrupulous dictators to produce a class of superior human beings. The same techniques could be also used in precisely the opposite way, to produce human-like creatures who would willingly perform the least-attractive and the most-dangerous work for a society. According to this view, Aldous Huxley's *Brave New World* should be updated, for modern molecular biology provides tyrants with tools for modifying human beings that Huxley could not have imagined in 1932.

The eighth and final argument against germ-line genetic intervention is raised chiefly by several European authors who place this argument in the context of human rights.[52] According to these commentators, human beings have a moral right to receive from their parents a genetic patrimony that has not been subjected to artificial tampering. Although the term "tampering" is not usually defined, it seems to mean any intentional effort to introduce genetic changes into the germ line, even if the goal is to reduce the likelihood that a genetic disease will be passed on to the children and grandchildren of a particular couple. The asserted right to be protected against such tampering may be a slightly different formulation of the sixth argument noted above—namely, that there are built-in limits, embedded in the nature of things, beyond which not even the most benevolent human beings should attempt to go.

A Brief Evaluation of the Arguments

In our view, the effort to cure and prevent serious disease and premature death is one of the noblest of all human undertakings. For this reason the first pro argument—that germ-line intervention may be the only way to treat or prevent certain diseases—seems to us to be of overriding importance. We also find the third pro argument to be quite strong, that a germ line correction, if demonstrated to be safe and effective, would be more efficient than repeated applications of somatic cell gene therapy. In addition, the final pro argument about the overall mission of the health professions and about society's approach to disabilities seems to us to provide a convincing justification for the germ-line approach, when gene replacement is available.

Our replies to the objections raised by critics of germ line intervention are as follows:

1. *Irreversible mistakes*. While we acknowledge that mistakes may be made in germ-line gene therapy, we think that the same sophisticated techniques that were employed to introduce the new genes will be able to be used to remove those genes or to compensate for their presence in some other way. Further, in any sphere of innovative therapy, a first step into human beings must be taken at some point.
2. *Alternative strategies*. Some couples, perhaps even most couples, will choose the alternative strategies of selective abortion or selective discard. In our view, a strategy of attempting to prevent or treat potential disease or disability in the particular biological individual accords more closely with the mission of the health sciences and shows greater respect for children and adults who are afflicted with disease or disability.
3. *High cost, limited availability*. It is too early to know what the relative cost of germ-line intervention will be when the technique is fully developed. In addition, the financial costs and other personal and social harms of preventable diseases will need to be compared with the financial costs of germ-line gene therapy. It is at least possible that this new technology could become widely diffused and available to many members of society.
4. *Use for enhancement*. Prudent social policy should be able to set limits on the use of germ-line genetic intervention. Further, some enhancements of human capabilities may be morally justifiable, especially when those enhancements are health related. We acknowledge that the distribution of genetic enhancement is an important question for policy makers. (The issue of enhancement is discussed in greater detail in the next chapter.)
5. *Human embryos*. In our view, research with early human embryos that is directed toward the development of germ-line gene therapy is morally justifi-

able in principle. Further, we acknowledge the potential of a totipotential cell but think that the value of a genetic diagnosis outweighs the value of such a cell. We also accept that, if a serious error is made in germ-line gene therapy, terminating the life of the resulting embryo or fetus may be morally justifiable. In short, there is a presumption in favor of fostering the continued development of human embryos and fetuses, but that presumption can in our view be overridden by other considerations like serious harm to the developing individual or others and the needs of preclinical research.

6. *Concentration of power*. We acknowledge that those who are able to use germ-line intervention will have unprecedented ability to introduce precise changes into the germ lines of particular individuals and families. However, in our view, it is better for human beings to possess this ability and to use it for constructive purposes like preventing disease in families than not to possess the ability. The central ethical question is public accountability by the scientists, health providers, and companies that will be involved with germ-line intervention. Such accountability presupposes transparency about the use of the technology and an ongoing monitoring process aimed at preventing its misuse.

7. *Misuse by dictators*. This objection focuses too much attention on technology and too little on politics. There is no doubt that bona fide tyrants have existed in the 20th century and that they have made use of all manner of technologies—whether the low-tech methods of surgical sterilization or the annihilation of concentration camp inmates with poison gas or high-tech weapons like nuclear warheads and long-range missiles—to terrify and to dominate. However, the best approach to preventing the misuse of genetic technologies may not be to discourage the development of the technologies but rather to preserve and encourage democratic institutions that can serve as an antidote to tyranny. A second possible reply to the tyrannical misuse objection is that germ-line intervention requires a long lead time, in order to allow the offspring produced to grow to adulthood. Tyrants are often impatient people and are likely to prefer the more instantaneous methods of propaganda, intimidation, and annihilation of enemies to the relatively slow pace of germ-line modification.

8. *Human rights and tampering*. It is a daunting task to imagine what the unborn and as-yet-unconceived generations of people coming after us will want.[53] Even more difficult is the effort to ascribe rights to human beings. Insofar as we can anticipate the needs and wants of future generations, we think that any reasonable future person would prefer health to serious disease and would therefore welcome a germ-line intervention in his or her family line that effectively prevented cystic fibrosis from being transmitted to him or her. In our view, such a person would not regard this intervention as tampering and would regard as odd the claim that his or her genetic patrimony has been artificially tampered with. Cystic fibrosis was not a part of his or her family's heritage that the future person was eager to receive or to claim.

Would Germ-Line Gene Therapy Be, or Lead to, a Eugenics Program?

We can perhaps best approach this question by imagining a future world in which the global elimination of a genetic disease by means of germ-line gene therapy is technically feasible.

The year is 2055, and a definitive genetic cure for the mutations that cause cystic fibrosis (CF) has recently been discovered, tested, and perfected. This target-specific mode of gene therapy takes a properly functioning gene to the site of the mutation, splices out and destroys the malfunctioning gene, and replaces it with the properly functioning gene. The new technique can be applied equally well to somatic and germ-line (sperm or egg) cells.

The World Health Organization (WHO) has recently announced a global program to eradicate all CF mutations from the human gene pool. The program is modeled on the earlier campaign to eliminate smallpox. All at-risk persons will be required to undergo testing and, if found to be affected or heterozygous, to accept genetic treatment of both their somatic and reproductive cells. WHO estimates that the global campaign will succeed within 35 years, at the most, and that the effort, when completed, will save $40 billion annually (in 2050 dollars) in the world health budget.

This hypothetical situation is extrapolated from past and present programs aimed at controlling serious infectious diseases. These programs include the worldwide campaign that eliminated smallpox, as well as state-based programs of mandatory immunization against such diseases as measles and polio.

A first issue raised by this hypothetical is whether it is reasonable to draw an analogy between infectious disease and genetic disease. Proponents of the analogy point to the transmissibility of disease in both cases and argue that the mere direction or mode of transmission—horizontal or vertical—is less important than the spread of disease. Opponents of the analogy point out that, while some infectious diseases are transmitted by intimate behavior, all genetic disease transmission occurs in the context of reproduction, one of the most intensely personal and private spheres of human life.

Second, we are not told in the hypothetical whether a voluntary program of genetic screening and gene therapy for CF has been tried and has failed. If it has not been tried, the burden of proof for the proponent of a mandatory program is heavier. Yet there may be plausible arguments, based on cost or the number of decades required to reach the goal in a voluntary program, for the moral preferability of the mandatory approach in this case and all relevantly similar cases. If a voluntary program has been tried and has failed because of public inertia or unreasonable resistance, a mandatory program might seem to be morally justifiable in this case, even to a civil libertarian, as a reasonable means to a highly desirable end.

Here we as coauthors see no alternative to drawing a sharp, clear moral and public-policy line. In our view, state intervention in reproductive decisions by individuals and couples is virtually always wrong and virtually always counterproductive as a public policy. We would apply this strong preference for voluntary public-health programs to several current technologies, for example, maternal serum alpha-fetoprotein screening to detect neural tube disorders, prenatal testing of HIV-infected pregnant women and postnatal testing of their infants, and newborn screening for genetic disease.[54] In the same way we would apply this preference to the future hypothetical possibility of germ-line genetic intervention. Thus, we would support the *offering* of diagnostic testing and germ-line gene therapy to all adults. In our view, the vast majority of individuals and couples would eagerly participate in such a program, just as the vast majority of parents consent to newborn testing in states where free choice in this matter is respected.[55] However, we regard state intervention to compel people to accept germ-line genetic intervention in their reproduction as a violation of a basic human right.

Would a voluntary germ-line program that aimed to reduce the incidence of one or more genetic diseases in human populations be a eugenics program? Much depends on whether the term *eugenics* is employed as a morally neutral, descriptive term or as term that already includes in its very meaning a negative moral judgment, like the words "murder" and "rape." The coercive and discriminatory eugenics programs adopted in the United States and Nazi Germany in the first half of the 20th century are rightly condemned as immoral.[56] The question remains, however, whether there is a place for the notion of a morally justifiable eugenics program—one that is strictly voluntary and firmly based on reliable genetic technologies. In our view, the word "eugenics" has been so tainted by the discriminatory, coercive practices of multiple nations in this century that it cannot be rehabilitated. Thus, we would want to use a different and probably more cumbersome formulation to describe such a program, for example, "a voluntary program to reduce the incidence of genetic disease through germ-line genetic intervention."

Finally, we note that the kind of public-health program outlined in this scenario would only be feasible if safe, reliable methods for effecting precise genetic changes in human sperm (or sperm-producing) cells and human egg cells within the bodies of adults are developed. Any technique that depends on in vitro fertilization and in vitro gene repair will be much too expensive to be used on a population-wide basis.

The Continuing Relevance of the "Points to Consider" and General Ethical Principles

The preceding chapter on somatic cell gene therapy discussed seven questions that are currently asked by the NIH RAC as it reviews somatic cell proposals. These questions are contained in a guidance document called the "Points to Consider."[57] The questions can be summarized as follows:

1. What is the disease to be treated?
2. What alternative treatments are available?
3. What is the potential harm of the intervention?
4. What is the potential benefit of the intervention?
5. How will the selection of patients be conducted in a way that is fair to all candidates?
6. How will the voluntary and informed consent of patients (or their parents or guardians) be solicited?
7. How will the privacy and confidentiality of patients be preserved?

In our view, these questions will be relevant to germ-line gene therapy proposals, but their emphasis will shift in important ways. In answering question 2, future researchers may need to discuss not only alternative *treatments* but also alternative strategies to prevent the transmission of genetic disorders to future generations. The options of preimplantation diagnosis and selective discard and of prenatal diagnosis and selective abortion will surely be discussed in this context. Questions 3 and 4 will also be pertinent but with an important shift in emphasis. If germ-line gene therapy is performed on early human embryos, the principal risks will be to the embryo and the embryo's potential descendants, not to the genetic parents of the embryo. Even if the parents have their sperm and egg cells treated in vivo by means of gene therapy, it is more likely that something will go wrong in the offspring than in the parents themselves. Similarly, the benefits of germ-line intervention will accrue primarily to the genetically repaired embryo and the embryo's future children rather than to the parents. Thus, the focus of the benefit–harm calculus will be expanded to include multiple future generations within a particular family, and both parents and researchers will know that their decisions will have long-term genetic effects.

The third and fourth questions will be broadened in another respect, as well. Some critics of germ-line genetic intervention have raised ethical objections to *ever* employing this technique on grounds of the serious social harm that might ensue. While the same critics have also been concerned about somatic cell gene therapy, their principal focus has been germ-line approaches.[58] Thus, researchers proposing to undertake germ-line gene therapy, or at least the review bodies evaluating such proposals, will need to take into account a much broader range of nonmedical consequences.[59]

Public and Expert Opinion on Germ-Line Gene Therapy

In the United States public opinion on germ-line gene therapy was sampled by the Louis Harris organization in 1986 and 1992.[60] Two types of questions were asked: one type focused on the disorders that children might inherit; the other explicitly asked about one-generation vs. multigenerational effects.

Table 3-5. Opinions about Specific Applications of Human Cell Manipulation

How do you feel about scientists changing the makeup of human cells? Would you strongly approve, somewhat approve, somewhat disapprove, or strongly disapprove for the indications listed below?[61]

	Strongly Approve	Somewhat Approve	Somewhat Disapprove	Strongly Disapprove	Not Sure
Stop [Prevent] children from inheriting a usually fatal genetic disease . . .	52% (51)	32% (33)	6% (8)	7% (7)	3% (1)
Stop [Prevent] children from inheriting a nonfatal birth defect [disease]	28% (41)	38% (36)	18% (12)	14% (9)	3% (2)

1992 vs. (1986)

Table 3-5 shows the first question, with the 1992 wording of the question noted in brackets and the 1986 percentages of respondents noted in parentheses.

In order to be sure that the subtlety of the word "inherited" did not escape the attention of respondents to a telephone interview, the 1986 Harris survey posed an explicit question about attitudes toward the germ-line approach. The question and responses are shown in Table 3-6.

On the basis of these two surveys, we can conclude that in 1986 a cross section of the general public, by a majority of about 75% to about 20%, accepted the germ-line approach to gene therapy in principle. Asked in a more subtle way about preventing the inheritance of disease by means of gene therapy, between 66% and 84% of respondents either strongly approved or somewhat approved, depending on the severity of the disease described in the question. Thus, it seems clear that substantial majority of the U.S. public is open to the possibility of germ-line gene therapy as a matter of general policy.

International expert opinion on germ-line genetic intervention is more evenly divided. All of the 28 policy statements on gene therapy cited in chapter 2 accept somatic cell approaches to gene therapy, but most expressed grave reservations

Table 3-6. Using Germ Line Versus Somatic Cells in Gene Therapy

Suppose someone had a genetic defect that would cause usually fatal diseases in them and would likely be inherited by their children. Do you think that doctors should be allowed to correct only the gene affecting the disease in the patient, only the gene that would carry the disease to future generations, both genes, or neither gene?[62]

	Both	Only Affecting Patient	Offspring	Neither	Not Sure
Total (1,273)	62%	8%	14%	11%	5%

about germ-line techniques. Typical of this position was a statement that emerged from a July 1979 conference sponsored by the World Council of Churches.

[W]e register opposition to the use of genetic engineering on the human fertilized ovum for purposes other than the correction of genetic defects, and even here we recommend that the research not proceed without full participation of the public in decisions of what is and what is not ethically acceptable in these procedures.[63]

The earliest government policy statement to discuss the germ-line question in detail was Recommendation 934 (1982) on genetic engineering, adopted by the European Parliamentary Assembly. With the memory of the Nazis' discriminatory and murderous eugenics programs still fresh in their minds, the European parliamentarians forthrightly asserted a human right to have a genome that has not been tampered with.[64] Yet, other parts of Recommendation 934 seemed to advocate the creation of a list of bona fide serious diseases (not including gender and race!) that would be legitimate targets for the germ-line approach.[65]

By the early 1990s policy statements on germ-line gene therapy seemed to reflect a greater openness to this future technological possibility. The clearest statement of support for the technique appeared in a 1990 statement of the Council for International Organizations of Medical Sciences (CIOMS). In the "Declaration of Inuyama" the delegates to an international meeting of the Council adopted the following recommendation about germ-line gene therapy:

VI. The modification of human germ cells for therapeutic or preventive purposes would be technically much more difficult than that of somatic cells and is not at present in prospect. However, such therapy might be the only means of treating certain conditions, and therefore continued discussion of both its technical and its ethical aspects is essential. Before germ-cell therapy is undertaken, its safety must be very well established, for changes in germ cells would affect the descendants of patients.[66]

Again, the results of public opinion polls and trends in expert opinion do not determine whether germ-line genetic intervention is morally right or wrong. At best, these surveys and policy statements provide supportive evidence for the moral judgments of others who have thought about this issue, either briefly or on a more sustained basis.

The Authors' Conclusion

Ultimately, the moral case for or against germ-line gene therapy must be established by good reasons. In our evaluation of the pro and con arguments and in our discussion of eugenics, we have attempted to indicate why we find voluntary programs of germ-line genetic intervention to be ethically acceptable in principle. We think that this strategy should be employed only when gene replacement or gene repair is a validated technique. In addition, we are hopeful that techniques will be developed for repairing sperm and egg cells in the bodies of prospective parents before fertilization occurs. Finally, we find both the goal of preventing disease in a particular individual and the goal of preventing the transmission of genetic disease to the individual's descendants to be worthy rationales for this intervention.

Where Should the Line Be Drawn?

In a widely cited article published in 1989, W. French Anderson advocated drawing the line between gene therapy aimed at curing or preventing disease, which he favored, and genetic intervention intended to enhance or improve the capacities of healthy human beings, which he opposed. According to Anderson, only this kind of line-drawing will focus the attention of gene therapy researchers on genuine *medical* problems, that is, on human disease and human health.[67]

Anderson may well be right in asserting that publicly funded agencies like the National Institutes of *Health* and researchers supported by public funds should give the highest priority to exploring new ways to combat life-threatening or severely disabling conditions that affect human beings. However, the ethical question remains: Is the use of genetic techniques to enhance human capabilities rather than to cure disease morally acceptable or unacceptable in general and in principle? We turn to this important question in our next chapter.

Notes

1. In fact, the Multiple Sclerosis Society has partially funded shiverer mice research. See Carol Readhead et al., "Expression of a Myelin Basic Protein Gene in Transgenic Shiverer Mice: Correction of the Dysmyelinating Phenotype," *Cell* 48(4): 711; 27 February 1987. Donald H. Silberg, "The Demyelinating Diseases," in James B. Wyngaarden et al. eds., *Cecil Textbook of Medicine* (2 vols.; 19th ed.; Philadelphia: W.B. Saunders, 1992), pp. 2196–2200.

2. Harold M. Schmeck, Jr., "Researchers Find More Genetic Clues to Multiple Sclerosis," *New York Times*, July 4, 1989, p. B2; Michael Waldholz, "New Research Links Multiple Sclerosis to the Inheritance of Certain Genes," *Wall Street Journal*, October 8, 1991, p. B10; Silberberg, op. cit.

3. The techniques they used were developed and described in Franklin Costantini and Elizabeth Lacy, "Introduction of Rabbit Beta-Globin into the Mouse Germ Line," *Nature* 294(5836): 92–94; 5 November 1981; and Jon W. Gordon et al., "Genetic Transformation of Mouse Embryos by Microinjection of Purified DNA," *Proceedings of the National Academy of Sciences* 77(12): 7380–7384; December 1980.

Hood and colleagues injected copies of the same DNA segment into zygotes from both shiverer and normal mice.

4. Readhead et al., op. cit., p. 704.

5. Ibid. The Hood team's meager yield is not unusual; the precarious processes of cell division, oviduct or uterine reimplantation, and embryo formation limit the number of zygotes that make it through the end of gestation even without having been the subject of genetic manipulation. Only 50–80% of mouse zygotes survive microinjection, and only

10–30% of the survivors develop to term after reimplantation. (In comparison, 60–70% of nonmicroinjected eggs survive implantation and develop to term.) (Personal communication with Frank Costantini [1983]. Transcript of the conference at Banbury Center, Cold Spring Harbor Laboratory, unedited version, "Prospects for Gene Therapy: Fact and Fiction," February 5–7, 1982, Session 2, pp. 68–69. See also Costantini and Lacy, op. cit.)

Hood and his team found that the only expressing transgenic mouse they had obtained had the normally occurring MBP alleles as well as the transgene. Unfortunately this did not allow them to study the effect of the transgene alone. Therefore, they crossed the transgenic mouse with homozygous shiverers to produce mice that had no normally occurring MBP genes but did have the transgene.

6. Readhead et al., pp. 704–705.

7. Readhead et al., pp. 703–712; Jon W. Gordon, "Transgenic Animals," *International Review of Cytology* 115:171–229; 1989; see p. 211.

8. See Gordon, pp. 210–212; and Richard D. Palmiter and Ralph L. Brinster, "Germ-Line Transformation of Mice," *Annual Review of Genetics* 20: 465–499, esp. 489–490; 1986; both articles collect examples of transgenic mice as models for gene therapy.

Frank Costantini and his colleagues corrected beta-thalassemia in mice in two different germ-line gene transfer experiments. In Costantini's first experiment, his team transferred a properly functioning beta-globin gene into the germ lines of thalassemic mice by microinjecting the gene into zygotes. The introduced beta-globin genes were properly regulated and tissue-specifically expressed, with the result that the mice's anemia was significantly reduced. In the second experiment, the team transferred a *human* beta-globin gene into the germ line of thalassemic mice, resulting in the complete elimination of the abnormalities in the mice's red blood cells that are associated with thalassemia. Researchers have attempted to achieve the same efficient expression of globin genes by somatic cell gene transfer into mouse bone-marrow stem cells with retroviral vectors, but without success. (Frank Costantini et al., "Correction of Murine Beta-Thalassemia by Gene Transfer into the Germ Line," *Science* 233[4769]: 1192–1194; 12 September 1986; see esp. p. 1192.)

Researchers at Genentech, Inc., have used germ-line gene transfer to restore reproductive functions in hypogonadal (hpg) mice. Hypogonadal mice have deletion mutations in a gene that encodes the biosynthetic precursor of gonadotropin-releasing hormone (GnRH). GnRH, a hormone released in the hypothalamus (a region of the brain), normally interacts with other hormones to promote sexual development and reproductive capacity. Lacking GnRH, hypogonadal mice are sexually immature, fail to develop mature germ cells, and are unable to reproduce. [Anthony J. Mason et al., "The Hypogonadal Mouse: Reproductive Functions Restored by Gene Therapy," *Science* 234(4782): 1372–1378; 12 December 1986.]

The Genentech researchers introduced the functioning GnRH gene into hypogonadal mice by first microinjecting the gene into normal mouse zygotes and then mating the resulting transgenic mice with heterozygous mice that carried hpg mutations. After two generations of matings, or crosses, the researchers were able to obtain mice that were homozygous for the hpg mutations (that is, both copies of the gene in each mouse were mutant) and also carried the GnRH transgene. This rather convoluted method of delivering the transgene to the germ line of hypogonadal mice was required because homozygous hypogonadal mice are infertile and cannot produce zygotes for microinjection. In fact, the practice of microinjecting healthy mice and then mating them with mice that carry a mutation is a common method of introducing transgenes into germ lines when direct microinjection is for some reason impractical. [Mason et al. (this endnote). For additional examples, see Costantini et al. (this endnote).]

The transgenic hypogonadal mice created by the Genentech researchers were sexually mature, able to mate and to become pregnant, and regained complete reproductive competence. Their littermates who did not receive the transgene remained developmentally arrested at the prepuberty stage. In addition, laboratory tests showed that the transgene was expressed in a tissue-specific manner in the mice who received it. [Mason, et al. (this endnote).]

Sly syndrome results from a deficiency in an enzyme called beta-glucuronosidase caused by a mutation in the gene for that enzyme. In both mice and humans, beta-glucuronosidase deficiency results in a chronic and progressive disease characterized by dwarfism, skeletal deformities, and premature death. Mice who have the equivalent of Sly syndrome are called *MPSVII mice.*

William Sly of Saint Louis University School of Medicine, and his research team, studied the effect of introducing a human gene for beta-glucuronidase into the germ line of MPSVII mice. They found that the MPSVII mice that received the human transgene expressed high levels of beta-glucuronosidase and were phenotypically normal, providing another example of complete correction of a disease in a mouse using a human gene. [John W. Kyle et al., "Correction of Murine Mucopolysaccharidosis VII by a Human Beta-Glucuronidase Transgene," *Proceedings of the National Academy of Sciences* 87(10): 3914–3918; May 1990.]

See also Catherine Cavard et al., "Correction of Mouse Ornithine Transcarbamylase Deficiency by Gene Transfer into the Germ Line," *Nucleic Acids Research* 16(5): 2099–2110; 25 March 1988; Torben Lund et al., "Prevention of Insulin-Dependent Diabetes Mellitus in Non-Obese Diabetic Mice by Transgenes Encoding Modified I-A Beta-Chain or Normal I-E Alpha-Chain," *Nature* 345(6277): 727–729; 21 June 1990; and J. Timothy Stout et al., "Expression of Human HPRT in the Central Nervous System of Transgenic Mice," *Nature* 317(6034): 250–252; 19 September 1985.

9. Ralph L. Brinster and Mary R. Avarbock, "Germline Transmission of Donor Haplotype Following Spermatogonial Transplantation," *Proceedings of the National Academy of Sciences* 91(24): 11301–11307; November 1994. See also the companion essay in the same issue of *PNAS*, Ralph L. Brinster and James W. Zimmerman, "Spermatogenesis Following Male Germ-Cell Transplantation," pp. 11298–11302. The quotation is from Brinster and Zimmerman, "Spermatogenesis," p. 11298.

10. Brinster and Zimmerman, op. cit., p. 11298.

11. Gina Kolata, *New York Times*, November 22, 1994, pp. A1, C10.

12. We define germ-line gene therapy according to the expected consequences of the techniques employed rather than according to the primary purpose of those techniques. This may create some confusion for students of the ethics of gene therapy. But it is necessary to acknowledge the dual effects of germ-line gene-therapy techniques that serve the primary purpose of treating a single patient and yet have germ-line alteration as an expected outcome. At least one of our critics has suggested separating categories of germ-line gene therapy according to the purposes of the strategies. While this approach may be useful for philosophers, it would make the categorization and evaluation of real-world gene-therapy proposals cumbersome. It would also necessitate an assessment of individual intent for each proposal rather than a review of expected outcomes.

13. See "The Declaration of Inuyama and Reports of the Working Groups," *Human Gene Therapy* 2(2): 123–129: Summer 1991; see esp. p. 129.

14. Ibid.

15. See Frank Fenner, *Smallpox and Its Eradication* (Geneva: World Health Organization, 1988); and United States, Congress, Office of Technology Assessment, *The Continuing Challenge of Tuberculosis* (Washington, DC: U.S. Government Printing Office, September 1993).

16. Robert C. King and William D. Stansfield, *A Dictionary of Genetics* (4th ed.; New York: Oxford University Press, 1990), p. 315. As a practical matter, totipotency is known to exist in human preembryos until at least the eight-cell stage. See A.H. Handyside, "Pregnancies from Biopsied Human Preimplantation Embryos Sexed by Y-specific DNA Amplification," *Nature* 344(6268): 768–770; 19 April 1990.

17. See pp. 61–62 above.

18. Handyside et al., "Pregnancies"; A.H. Handyside et al., "Biopsy of Human Preimplantation Embryos and Sexing by DNA Amplification," *Lancet* 1(8634): 347–349; 18 February 1989; and Peter Gorner and Ronald Kotulak, "Gene Screening: A Chance to Map Our Body's Future," *Chicago Tribune*, April 15, 1990, Section 1, p. 1.

19. Ron Winslow, "Hoffmann-La Roche to Ease Curb on Gene Technology," *Wall Street Journal*, January 27, 1992, p. B1.

20. Gordon, op. cit. (note 8), pp. 175, 176; George Scangos and Charles Bieberich, "Gene Transfer into Mice," *Advances in Genetics* 24: 285–322, esp. p. 287; 1987; Colin L. Stewart, et al., "Expression of Retroviral Vectors in Transgenic Mice Obtained by Embryo Infection," *EMBO Journal* 6(2): 383–388; February 1987; and Herman Van Der Putten et al., "Efficient Insertion of Genes into the Mouse Germ Line via Retroviral Vectors," *Proceedings of the National Academy of Sciences* 82(18): 6148–6152; September 1985.

21. Gordon, pp. 173–174; Scangos and Bieberich, p. 285; Moshe Shani, "Tissue-Specific and Developmentally Regulated Expression of a Chimeric Actin-Globin Gene in Transgenic Mice," *Molecular and Cellular Biology* 6(7): 2624–2631; July 1986; Costantini et al. (note 8); Richard N. Sifers et al., "Tissue Specific Expression of Human Alpha-1–Antitrypsin Gene in Transgenic Mice," *Nucleic Acids Research* 15(4): 1459–1475; 25 February 1987; K.H. Choo et al., "Expression of Active Human Blood Clotting Factor IX in Transgenic Mice: Use of a cDNA with Complete mRNA Sequence," *Nucleic Acids Research* 15(3): 871–874; 11 February 1987; and Costantini and Lacy (note 3).

22. Scangos and Bieberich (note 20), p. 290; Philippe Soriano et al., "Tissue-Specific and Ectopic Expression of Gene Introduced into Transgenic Mice by Retroviruses," *Science* 234(4782): 1409–1413; 12 December 1986.

23. Gordon (note 7), pp. 175–176.

24. Thomas M. DeChiara et al., "A Growth-Deficiency Phenotype in Heterozygous Mice Carrying an Insulin-Like Growth Factor II Gene Disrupted by Targeting," *Nature* 345(6270): 78–80; 3 May 1990; Randall S. Johnson et al., "Targeting of Nonexpressed Genes in Embryonic Stem Cells Via Homologous Recombination," *Science* 245(4923): 1234–1236; 15 September 1989; Mario R. Capecchi, "Altering the Genome by Homologous Recombination," *Science* 244(4910): 1288–1292; 16 June 1989; and Suzanne L. Mansour, "Disruption of the Proto-Oncogene *int-2* in Mouse Embryo-Derived Stem Cells: A General Strategy for Targeting Mutations to Non-Selectable Genes," *Nature* 336(6197): 348–352; 24 November 1988.

25. Marcia Barinaga, "Gene-Transfer Method Fails Test," *Science* 246(4929): 446; 27 October 1989.

26. See pp. 61–62 above.

27. It is possible that a gene, delivered as part of a vector that has its own origin of replication (that is, locus from which replication can begin), may effect gene therapy without integration. But gene transfer experiments in animals generally involve integrating genes.

28. *Webster's New Collegiate Dictionary* (Springfield, MA: G. & C. Merriam Company, 1973), p. 193.

29. King and Stansfield (note 16), p. 54.

30. Theoretically, germ-line transfer directly into gametes would result in genetically consistent individuals because the genetic alteration would be inherited by all of the resulting individual's cells. However, researchers have not yet developed techniques that successfully deliver genes into fully differentiated gametes. Brinster and his colleagues have succeeded in transplanting mouse sperm stem cells. See pp. 61–62.

31. Carol Ezzell, "Sheep Chimera Makes Human Blood Cells," *Science News* 141(12): 182; 21 March 1992.

32. Frank Costantini, Gene Therapy Lecture for Medical Genetics 1015, Columbia University (March 15, 1983); Capecchi (note 24).

33. In theory, it would be possible, however, to add a gene whose product specifically inactivated the inappropriate gene product of a dominant genetic disease and thereby to treat a dominant disease with gene addition. There does not appear to be much activity in this area in the scientific literature.

34. Oliver Smithies et al., "Insertion of DNA Sequences into the Human Chromosomal Beta-Globin Locus by Homologous Recombination," *Nature* 317(6034): 230–234; 19 September 1985; Johnson et al. (note 24); Mansour et al. (note 24).

35. John C. Fletcher and W. French Anderson, "Germ-Line Gene Therapy: A New Stage of Debate," *Law, Medicine, and Health Care* 20(1–2): 26–39; Spring-Summer 1992; see esp. p. 13. See also Handyside et al., "Pregnancies" (note 18).

36. Two recent discussions of this topic are Ronald Munson and Lawrence Davis, "Germ-Line Gene Therapy and the Medical Imperative," *Kennedy Institute of Ethics Journal* 2(2): 137–158; June 1992; and Nelson A. Wivel and LeRoy Walters, "Germ-Line Gene Modification and Disease Prevention: Some Medical and Ethical Perspectives," *Science* 262(5133): 533–538; 22 October 1993.

37. See especially J.B.S. Haldane, *Daedalus, or Science and the Future* (New York: E.P. Dutton & Company, 1924).

38. See especially H.J. Muller, *Out of the Night: A Biologist's View of the Future* (New York: Vanguard Press, 1935).

39. See H.J. Muller, "The Guidance of Human Evolution," *Perspectives in Biology and Medicine* 3(1): 1–43; Autumn 1959; see also Muller's "Human Evolution by Voluntary Choice of Germ Plasm," *Science* 134(3480): 643–649; 8 September 1961. An early book by Muller on this topic was *Out of the Night*; see esp. pp. 103–127. For a secondary account of Muller's views, see Elof Axel Carlson, *Genes, Radiation, and Society: The Life and Work of H.J. Muller* (Ithaca, NY: Cornell University Press, 1981), pp. 393–404.

40. Joshua Lederberg, "Biological Future of Man," in Gordon Wolstenholme, ed., *Man and His Future* (London: J. & A. Churchill, 1963), p. 265.

41. James V. Neel, "Germ-Line Gene Therapy: Another View," *Human Gene Therapy* 4(2): 127; April 1993.

42. It is perhaps worth noting that researchers performing somatic-cell gene therapy have carefully avoided diseases and subtypes of diseases that affect mental functioning. One thinks, for example, of Lesch-Nyhan syndrome, of certain subtypes of Gaucher disease and Hunter syndrome, of Tay-Sachs disease, and of metachromatic leukodystrophy.

43. We owe the suggestion of retinoblastoma as a candidate disorder to Kevin FitzGerald, S.J. We are also indebted to Nelson A. Wivel for information on the genetics of retinoblastoma. See Wivel and Walters (note 37). See also Stephen H. Friend et al., "A Human DNA Segment with Properties of the Gene That Predisposes to Retinoblastoma and Osteosarcoma," *Nature* 323(6089): 643–646; 16 October 1986; and Ei Matsunaga, "Hereditary Retinoblastoma: Host Resistance and Second Primary Tumors," *Journal of the National Cancer Institute* 65(1): 47–51; July 1980.

44. Although the genetics of the germ-line p53 gene mutation are more complex than the genetics of the germ-line mutation that causes retinoblastoma, p53 may turn out to be another important tumor suppressor gene to which the same comments apply. On the germ-line p53 mutation, see Frederick P. Li et al., "Recommendations on Predictive Testing for Germ LIne p53 Mutations Among Cancer-Prone Individuals," *Journal of the National Cancer Institute* 84(15): 1156–1160; 5 August 1992; and Curtis C. Harris and Monica Hollstein, "Clinical Implications of the *p53* Tumor-Suppressor Gene," *New England Journal of Medicine* 329(18): 1318–1327; 28 October 1993.

45. Eric T. Juengst, "Germ-Line Gene Therapy: Back to Basics," *Journal of Medicine and Philosophy* 16(6): 589–590; December 1991.

46. Burke K. Zimmerman, "Human Germ-Line Therapy: The Case for Its Development and Use," *Journal of Medicine and Philosophy* 16(6): 596–598; December 1991.

47. For a detailed discussion of and justification for germ-line intervention in this setting, see Marc Lappé, "Ethical Issues in Manipulating the Human Germ Line," *Journal of Medicine and Philosophy* 16(6): 621–639; December 1991.

48. As noted above (pp.), already in 1962 Joshua Lederberg was arguing against H.J. Muller's proposals for improving the human gene pool through programs of "voluntary germinal choice" by appealing to the prospect of rapid, global genetic intervention by means of germ-line gene therapy. See Joshua Lederberg, "Biological Future of Man," in Gordon Wolstenholme, ed., *Man and His Future* (London: J. & A. Churchill, 1963), pp. 265 and 269.

49. On the general issue of the freedom of scientific inquiry, see Loren R. Graham, "Concerns About Science and Attempts to Regulate Inquiry," *Daedalus* 107(2): 1–21; Spring 1978.

50. National Institutes of Health, Human Embryo Research Panel, *Report* (Bethesda, MD: NIH, 27 September 1994).

51. See, for example, the following critiques of human embryo research: "The Inhuman Use of Human Beings," *First Things* 49: 17–21; January 1995; Dianne N. Irving, "Testimony before the NIH Human Embryo Research Panel," *Linacre Quarterly* 61(4): 82–89; November 1994; and Kevin O'Rourke, "Embryo Research: Ethical Issues," *Health Care Ethics USA* 2(4): 2–3; Fall 1994.

52. Mauron and Thévoz, op. cit.

53. There is a rather substantial literature on this topic. See, for example, Ruth Faden, Gail Geller, and Madison Powers, eds., *AIDS, Women and the Next Generation* (New York: Oxford University Press, 1991); LeRoy Walters, "Ethical Issues in Maternal Serum Alpha-Fetoprotein Testing and Screening: A Reappraisal," in Mark I. Evans et al., eds., *Fetal Diagnosis and Therapy: Science, Ethics and the Law* (Philadelphia: J.B. Lippincott, 1989), pp. 54–60; and Lori B. Andrews et al., eds., *Assessing Genetic Risks: Implications for Health and Social Policy: Report* (Washington, DC: National Academy Press, 1994).

54. On prenatal testing of HIV infected pregnant women see Faden, Geller, and Powers, eds., ibid. On newborn screening see Andrews et al., eds., op. cit.

55. See Ruth R. Faden et al., "A Survey to Evaluate Parental Consent as Public Policy for Neonatal Screening," *American Journal of Public Health* 72(12): 1347–1352; December 1982.

56. Philip R. Reilly, *The Surgical Solution* (Baltimore: Johns Hopkins University Press, 1991); Robert N. Proctor, *Racial Hygiene: Medicine under the Nazis* (Cambridge, MA: Harvard University Press, 1988).

57. U.S., National Institutes of Health, "Recombinant DNA Research: Actions under the Guidelines," *Federal Register* 60(81): 20726–20737; 27 April 1995.

58. Council for Responsible Genetics, "Position Paper on Human Germ Line Manipulation (Fall 1992)," *Human Gene Therapy* 4(1): 35–37; February 1993.

59. On the relevance of the "Points to Consider" to germ-line gene therapy, see the provocative essay by Eric T. Juengst, "The NIH 'Points to Consider' and the Limits of Human Gene Therapy," *Human Gene Therapy* 1(4): 425–433; Winter 1990.

60. See the fuller discussion of these two surveys in Chapter 2, p. 44. The first survey was taken for the Office of Technology Assessment in 1986, the second for the March of Dimes in 1992.

61. U.S., Congress, Office of Technology Assessment (OTA), *New Developments in Biotechnology—Background Paper: Public Perceptions of Biotechnology* (Washington, DC: U.S. Government Printing Office, May 1987), p. 73, Table 53; March of Dimes Birth Defects Foundation (MOD), "Genetic Testing and Gene Therapy Survey: Questionnaire and Responses," (White Plains, NY: March of Dimes Birth Defects Foundation, September 1992), p. 3, B3 c and d.

62. OTA (note 63), p. 74.

63. "Ethical Issues in the Biological Manipulation of Life," in Paul Abrecht, ed., *Faith and Science in an Unjust World: Report of the World Council of Churches' Conference on Faith, Science and the Future*, Vol. 2: *Reports and Recommendations* (Philadelphia: Fortress Press, 1980), pp. 49–68; here, p. 66.

64. Council of Europe, Parliamentary Assembly, "Recommendation 934 (1982) on Genetic Engineering," adopted 26 January 1982, in *Texts Adopted by the Assembly*, 33rd Ordinary Session, Third Part, January 25–29, 1982 (Strasbourg: the Council, 1982).

65. Ibid.

66. "Declaration of Inuyama" (note 13), p. 129.

67. W. French Anderson, "Human Gene Therapy: Why Draw a Line?" *Journal of Medicine and Philosophy* 14(6): 681–693; December 1989.

4

Enhancement
Genetic
Engineering

Scientific Issues

Imagine the results of adding a size-enhancing gene to the genome of a short person. Such visions are not far-fetched. Indeed, in a series of studies, researchers Richard D. Palmiter, Ralph L. Brinster, Robert E. Hammer, and their colleagues have produced spectacular results by inserting various forms of a growth-stimulating gene into mouse germ lines using microinjection[1] (Figure 4–1).

The gene inserted by Palmiter and his colleagues encoded a protein called *growth hormone*, a key hormone in both humans and mice. In one study, the researchers microinjected into fertilized mouse eggs a rat growth hormone gene that had been fused to a regulatory element of another gene, the *metallothionein gene promoter*. The fusion of the rat growth hormone gene to this distinctive promoter allowed the researchers to regulate the expression of the *fusion gene* in vivo by administering heavy metals to the mice. When they administered heavy metals to the mice, they induced expression of the fusion gene and thus, the production of growth hormone. The transgenic mice produced by this study exhibited dramatic growth and were significantly larger than their nonengineered counterparts.[2]

Similar experiments by Palmiter, Brinster, and Hammer, using the *human* growth hormone gene and a related human growth factor, spawned similar gigantism in mice.[3] Moreover, the researchers demonstrated by breeding these transgenic mice that the characteristic of rapid growth can be inherited by mice who inherit a growth hormone transgene.[4]

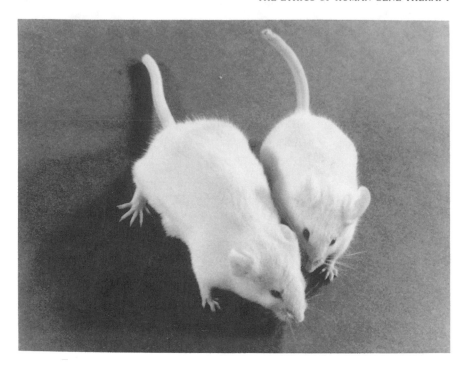

Figure 4–1. Two male mice from Palmiter et al.'s genetic engineering experiments. The mouse on the left contains a new gene composed of the mouse metallothionein promoter fused to the rat growth hormone structural gene. The gene is passed on to offspring which also grow larger than controls. Source: Dr. R. L. Brinster, professor of physiology in the Department of Animal Biology at the School of Veterinary Medicine, University of Pennsylvania.

Although these experiments illustrated immense potential for genetic enhancement of size, they also revealed the flaws in current techniques. For instance, many of the transgenic giant mice were infertile, and some suffered from cancerous tumors.[5] Many defects in scientific methodology remain to be resolved before genetic enhancements will be risk-free, but the technological ability to genetically enhance certain human characteristics steadily approaches.

Gene transfer technologies, both somatic cell and germ line, someday will be applicable for enhancement purposes, just as surgical methods developed for treating human health disorders are used currently for cosmetic enhancements. However, as has often been pointed out, the use of genetic engineering for human enhancement should not be expected at any time in the near future, for many reasons, including the high level of complexity of most of the traits people would like to enhance.[6] Thus, the descriptions of the scientific aspects of enhancement engineering in this chapter, while not science fiction, are somewhat futuristic.

In addition to size, genetic enhancement has been contemplated, with varying degrees of seriousness, for traits such as intelligence, memory, sleep dependence, aggression, kindness, aging, gender, and other behavioral and personality characteristics.[7] Many of these traits are difficult to define, measure or quantify, and all of them are believed to be multifactorial. That is, they are determined by many complex factors, most likely including more than one gene in addition to environmental components. The technologies necessary for tackling such traits presently elude researchers. One factor that makes the directed alteration of multifactorial traits difficult is the complexity of the genetic regulation required to coordinate the expression of several genes in conjunction with environmental influences.

Another factor is the difficulty of pinning down the phenotype for any particular multifactorial trait. In describing research advances in the genetics of hypertension, one author noted that even quantitative traits like a person's blood pressure vary throughout the day and are therefore difficult to pinpoint precisely. This problem is even more pronounced with respect to personality and behavioral characteristics, such as intelligence and aggression. Finding genes that contribute to these characteristics requires first establishing an objective definition of the characteristics, an enigmatic task. Before researchers look for the genetic determinants of a trait such as aggressiveness, they must be able to accurately and objectively identify aggressive individuals. Accurate identification of aggressive individuals is made extremely difficult by the mercurial manner in which the trait of aggressiveness is displayed. Linking such difficult-to-define traits with genes must be approached with caution because one is never sure whether the trait really exists in the person in question.[8]

Potential Enhancements

Despite the difficulties associated with complex gene regulation and the definition of personality and behavioral phenotypes, recent research advances have boosted the prospects for enhancement genetic engineering. Five potential types of enhancements, presented below, together with the research results that support them, are particularly compelling examples of the prospects for enhancement genetic engineering.

Size. An often-cited example of prospective enhancement engineering is increased height, or stature. Human stature is determined by, among other things, the biological availability of human growth hormone, a key growth-stimulating protein. The human growth hormone gene has therefore been the subject of much enhancement-gene-therapy speculation.[9]

Growth hormone gene therapy can be envisioned as a somatic cell gene therapy or as a germ-line gene therapy. The Palmiter, Brinster, and Hammer research in mice, described at the beginning of this chapter, suggests that the germ-line insertion of a growth hormone gene could enhance the stature of a child who is otherwise destined to be short, or even average in size. However, all of the technical obstacles to human germ-line gene therapy similarly impede germ-line gene enhancement of stature.

The prospective success of somatic-cell growth-hormone gene transfer might be extrapolated from the results of somatic cell administration of the hormone itself. Human growth hormone (GH) has been administered directly to both GH-deficient children (who can be classified as having a disorder) and to short, non–GH-deficient children (who are otherwise healthy), with some reported success.[10] If hormone administration proves consistently successful in promoting increased stature, then transferring the gene encoding that hormone into a patient's cells, where it will encode the production of growth hormone in vivo, can be expected to achieve the same goal.

Sleep. In January 1993, the United States National Commission on Sleep Disorders Research issued a report which concluded that sleepiness, caused by sleep disorders or simple lack of sleep, imposes devastating social and economic costs on American society. For example, the commission reported that at least two recent catastrophes—the 1989 *Exxon Valdez* oil spill in Alaska and the 1979 Three Mile Island nuclear plant accident—could be attributed to fatigue due to workers' lack of sleep. The commission also warned that sleep problems are responsible for numerous highway and workplace accidents resulting in loss of life and billions of dollars in lost productivity, medical costs, and sick leaves per year.[11] On a daily basis, millions of Americans, including fighter pilots, medical residents, travelers suffering from jet lag, spouses of snorers, and parents of newborns, struggle to function effectively on inadequate sleep. It would not be surprising, therefore, if demand arose for a genetic method to reduce the need for sleep.

Sleep research has indicated that our sleep cycles and even our need for sleep are controlled, at least in part, by proteins in our brains. Researchers have discovered a master neurological timer called the *suprachiasmatic nucleus*, located in the brain's hypothalamus. This timer has also been called the *circadian clock*.[12] This region regulates daily cycles such as sleepiness, hormone levels, and body temperature. In 1992, Joseph S. Takahashi and his co-workers at Northwestern University in Evanston, Illinois, reported that two genes, called *c-fos* and *jun-B*, together stimulate the production of a protein called AP-1 transcription factor, which may be involved in resetting the circadian clock. They kept hamsters in complete darkness for several days before exposing them to a brief burst of light. They found "an extremely tight correlation between the effects of light on the [circadian] clock and its resetting, and the effects of light on the genes and AP-1."[13]

These interesting results have been verified through additional research. For example, more recent studies by Takahashi and his colleagues have discovered a mutation called *Clock* in mice; for mice that are homozygous for this mutation, the average "day" was 27–28 hours long.[14] Already in the late 1980s, Seymour Benzer of Caltech and his colleagues had found a clock gene called *per*, or *period*, in the fruit fly.[15] Many years earlier, in March 1981, researchers Miodrag Radulovacki and colleagues had shown that the administration of either one of two pharmacological agents, phenoxybenzamine or bromocriptine, to rats immediately before or during sleep deprivation fulfilled the need for sleep in the rats and abolished the symptoms of sleep deprivation.[16] These studies suggest that genes and brain chemicals can alter sleep cycles and the actual need for sleep.

If these results hold true in humans as well as animals, one could imagine a somatic genetic enhancement involving cell grafting in the hypothalamus designed to reduce an individual's need for sleep.[17] In this hypothetical scenario, a gene for an agent that could reset the circadian clock or reduce the need for sleep would be transferred to cells that could be implanted in the hypothalamus. There they would cooperate with the brain cells controlling sleep. This presumes that regulation of the transferred genes could somehow be preset or controlled in vivo. Implementing such an enhancement in the germ line would, of course, be far more complicated. And who would take on the difficult task of raising the resulting child whose need for sleep had been reduced? Perhaps the only qualified people would be parents who had received somatic genetic enhancement that reduced their own need for sleep.

Aging. Since the time when adventurers searched for the "fountain of youth," explorers have probed for a way to slow down aging. Genetic engineering may ultimately provide the key to prolonged youth. In August 1990, researcher Thomas E. Johnson, of the University of Colorado, reported his studies of mutant nematodes (a type of roundworm) that experienced a significant increase in life span as a result of their genetic mutation.[18] The long-lived nematodes had a mutation in a single gene, labeled the *age-1* gene, and lived 40–60% longer than average.[19] Studies of the life-prolonging mutation in nematodes convinced Johnson that it may one day be possible to modify the speed of the aging process in humans.[20]

Similar discoveries in fruit flies and yeast support the notion that the human life-span may someday be increased through genetic enhancement.[21] Evolutionary biologist Michael Rose reported at the 1992 annual meeting of the American Association for the Advancement of Science that he and his research team had increased the life-spans of fruit flies, yeast, and roundworms by manipulating genes. Rose and colleagues worked with an anti-aging gene that encodes an enzyme called *superoxide dismutase (SOD)*. SOD counteracts *free radicals*, particles that can wreak havoc on cells by causing frequent small disruptions in their DNA. Much of the damage caused by free radicals is repaired by regular DNA repair systems inherent in the cells. But over time, some of the damage eludes repair and cells suffer the gradual decline we call aging. Mutations which make the SOD gene more active allow cells to better protect their DNA from free radical damage, and thus from the effects of advanced age.

Rose and Johnson both believe that "there is a real possibility of affecting the aging process with biomedical intervention."[22] Johnson has speculated that genetic manipulation involving the insertion of hyperactive human SOD genes into bone marrow stem cells might provide an anti-aging "therapy."[23]

Evidence that human aging, like aging in nematodes and fruit flies, is under genetic control is provided by a recent study that localized to a single chromosomal region the gene responsible for an aging disease called *Werner syndrome*. Japanese researcher Makoto Goto and others (including scientists at the American company Genentech) studied 21 families that had members who suffered from this rare genetic disease in which the affected individuals age prematurely.[24] Although Werner syndrome is a clinically complex disease affecting all tissues of the body in a way that resembles normal aging, Goto and colleagues were persuaded by their study that a single gene is probably responsible for the disease. It is possible that future studies of the gene responsible for Werner's syndrome will provide insights into normal aging in humans and will lead to genetic strategies for enhancing human life-spans.

Memory. The ability to remember words, names, facts, and experiences is one thing many people might like to improve for themselves and their offspring. It is generally agreed that human memory is a phenomenon that occurs in the brain through the transfer of chemicals from one brain cell to another. When certain *transmitter* chemicals are released from a nerve cell in the brain, they are received by receptors on the surface of other, neighboring nerve cells. One such receptor, called N-methyl-D-aspartate (NMDA), has been the subject of several studies. Together, these studies have established that the NMDA receptor, upon contact with a neurotransmitter called *glutamate*, "opens" and becomes a channel for positively charged calcium atoms, thereby initiating the conduction of an electrical impulse along the nerve cell (Figure 4-2). Such nerve cell impulses are the biological basis for at least some aspects of the phenomenon of memory. It has been suggested that an increase in the number of NMDA receptors, an increase in the sensitivity of NMDA receptors, or an increase in the amount of the transmitters received by NMDA receptors might enhance memory.[25]

In November 1991, Japanese researcher Koki Moriyoshi and others reported their identification of the gene that encodes the NMDA receptor in rats.[26] In the same issue of the journal *Nature*, researchers Keshava N. Kumar of the University of Kansas and others reported their cloning of the gene that encodes the NMDA subunit responsible for binding to glutamate.[27] The identifications of the NMDA gene and the gene for one of its most critical subunits were triumphs for the field of brain biology, and perhaps moved researchers one step closer to achieving the ability to manipulate memory with the tools of genetic engineering. One can imagine scenarios in which somatic cell gene transfer (perhaps via cell grafting, because current technologies do not allow nerve cells to be removed and then reintroduced

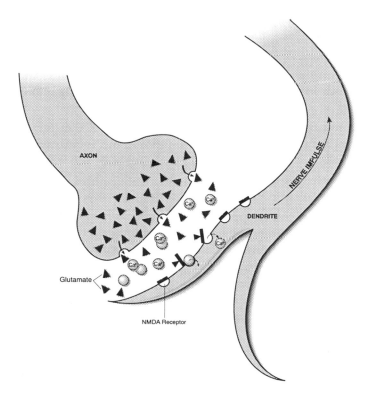

Figure 4–2. NMDA receptors.

into the human body) or germ-line gene transfer (that is, early embryo or gamete gene transfer) could be used to improve human memory. The enhancement would be carried out by inserting NMDA genes into human cells either to increase the number of NMDA receptors in brain cells or to improve the sensitivity of the receptors.[28]

The striking success of human studies in which memory has been facilitated by the administration of drugs affecting NMDA receptors suggests that there is great potential for human genetic memory enhancements. Certain chemicals facilitate the interaction of the NMDA receptor with glutamate. One such chemical is *glycine*, which, in the presence of a form of glutamate, increases the likelihood that the NMDA receptor will open into a channel for calcium. A 1991 study by Barbara L. Schwartz of the Veterans Administration Medical Center and the Georgetown University School of Medicine, and her colleagues, demonstrated that a drug called *milacemide*, which is converted in vivo to glycine, enhances human memory in both young and old normal adults. In their study Schwartz and colleagues gave human subjects definitions of various words and asked them to retrieve from their memories the name of the defined word. For example, subjects might read "bits of colored paper scattered at festive occasions." The target word to be retrieved from memory then would be "confetti." Subjects performed the word retrieval tasks on consecutive days after receiving either milacemide or a placebo. The researchers found that milacemide administration improved the word retrieval performance of study subjects.[29] This finding has implications for genetic enhancements of human memory, because it suggests that a genetic alteration that caused increased production of a milacemide-like molecule might facilitate the opening of NMDA channels and thereby enhance human memory.

Another research advance presages the ability to better understand the genetic components of human memory and may one day lead to genetic enhancement of memory. Researchers have recently identified the genetic mutations associated with two distinct hereditary forms of Alzheimer disease (AD).[30] One form of hereditary AD afflicts patients in their early 40s with the onset of short-term-memory problems and a gradual progression to other cognitive difficulties.[31] Mutations in the amyloid precursor gene on chromosome 21 are associated with this disorder in some families; however, the majority of cases seem to be linked to chromosome 14, although the precise gene has not yet been identified.[32] In 1993 the genetic locus responsible for about 17% of late-onset AD in the United States was identified. This locus on chromosome 19 is called apolipoprotein E. One variant at this locus, called *Apo*-E4, is associated with a higher-than-average risk for late-onset AD. In fact, people who have one or two copies of the *Apo*-E4 allele are more than six times as likely to develop late-onset AD as those who have none.[33]

Aggression. Aggression is often cited as an example of a prime candidate for genetic manipulation, although it is not clear whether the desired change would be an increase or decrease in aggressive tendencies.[34] An indication that a complex behavioral characteristic like aggression might have manipulable genetic determinants can be found in research on Lesch-Nyhan syndrome.

As described in Chapter 2, Lesch-Nyhan syndrome is a tragic disease associated with behavioral abnormalities, including aggressive self-mutilation.[35] A defect in a single gene is responsible for Lesch-Nyhan syndrome, causing all of the symptoms of the disease including the behavior of self-mutilation. That a single genetic mutation causes such a complex and peculiar behavior is powerful support for the concept that certain behavioral traits may be specified by single genes or simple combinations of genes. If researchers could identify genes responsible for other aggressive tendencies, besides self-mutilation, it is possible that genetic alterations could augment or reduce these tendencies.

In fact, researchers have used germ-line gene transfer to correct the mouse equivalent of Lesch-Nyhan syndrome.[36] Although the diseased mice did not suffer from the behavioral abnormalities that plague human Lesch-Nyhan syndrome patients, the success in correcting the disease in mice may indicate that it will one day be possible to correct Lesch-Nyhan syndrome in humans, including its behavioral components.

Researchers have been able to influence the aggressive behavior of laboratory animals by both classical and molecular genetic techniques. For example, high- and low-aggressive populations of mice and foxes have been developed, through repeated selection, in both species.[37] In addition, a researcher from the Institut National de la Santé et de la Recherche Médicale (INSERM) in Strasbourg, France—René Hen—has used *knockout* techniques with mice—techniques that inactivate the gene for one type of receptor for serotonin, a neurotransmitter. The resulting mice, with lower-than-normal levels of serotonin, displayed aggressive behavior toward other mice.[38]

In 1993 Dutch geneticists reported on a mutation that may be associated with impulsive, violent behavior in an extended family in the Netherlands. As discussed in more detail below, a mutation on the X chromosome in some members of this family interferes with the production of a single enzyme, monoamine oxidase A. This enzyme, in turn, seems to play a role in regulating the levels of serotonin and noradrenaline in the brain.[39] If the findings of the Dutch group are validated by further research, this mutation may provide one of the clearest examples of a pathway that leads from a gene to the nervous system to antisocial behavior.

These studies suggest that the genetic modification of behavioral characteristics like a tendency to aggression, whether disease-related or not, will perhaps one day be achievable.

General cognitive ability. The possible links between genes and general cognitive ability, sometimes called *intelligence*, cannot easily be studied in laboratory animals. Further, the validity of current methods for measuring human cognitive abilities and the reliability of existing evidence concerning the connection between genes and cognitive function are matters of some dispute. We will therefore consider both the scientific and the ethical dimensions of this controversial topic in the ethics section of the chapter.

Summary

Even with all of the knowledge researchers have accumulated thus far, many years of research remain before germ-line gene transfer for the purpose of enhancing memory, aggression, or aging will be feasible. Researchers have much to learn before they can use genetic engineering techniques to address complex human personality and behavioral traits. First, researchers must understand the precise biological basis for such traits and how that biology interacts with stimuli received from the outside environment. Nevertheless, the current pace of research suggests that complex traits like memory, aggression, and aging may one day be accessible to genetic intervention. Genetic enhancement of human stature may be technologically even closer.

Ethical Issues

Proponents of gene-mediated enhancement of human capabilities have generally distinguished three spheres in which such enhancements might be effected: (1) physical strength and longevity; (2) intelligence, or components of intelligence, including memory; and (3) attitudes toward, and behavior in relation to, one's fellow human beings. For the sake of simplicity we will designate these three types of conceivable enhancements *physical, intellectual,* and *moral.* We recognize, of course, that these conceptual distinctions are not always sharp and clear. We also acknowledge that, in even discussing these three kinds of enhancements by genetic means, we are tacitly accepting a genetic influence on (but not a genetic determination of) physical, intellectual, and even moral traits.[40]

Historical Background

The first statement to outline three spheres for possible human genetic enhancement was drafted by classical geneticist Hermann J. Muller during the Seventh International Congress of Genetics held in Edinburgh, Scotland, in August 1939. At that time, on the eve of World War II, Trofim Lysensko's ideological approach to genetics was already receiving strong support from Stalin, the Communist party chief in the U.S.S.R. Lysenko defied the available scientific evidence and asserted the Lamarckian doctrine that acquired traits could be passed on to one's descendants through the germ line. The Larmarckian view fit well with Marxist theory because it allowed the social changes advocated by the Communist party to have a genetic effect on the next generation.[41] At the same time, under Adolf Hitler the Nazi government of Germany had already implemented many discriminatory and brutal measures under its program of racial hygiene.[42] At the congress the participants were challenged by Science Service[43] to respond to the following question: "How could the world's population be improved most effectively genetically?"[44] The reply to this question, signed by 23 scientists, was popularly known as the "Geneticists' Manifesto." The manifesto by no means adopted the perspective of biological determinism. Rather, it accented both social and genetic changes that could enhance human well-being.

In the section of the manifesto devoted to genetic objectives, Muller wrote:

The most important genetic objectives, from a social point of view, are the improvement of those genetic characteristics which make for (a) health, (b) for the complex called intelligence, and (c) for those temperamental qualities which favour fellow-feeling and social behaviour rather than those (to-day most esteemed by many) which make for personal 'success', as success is usually understood at present.[45]

In 1959, the centennial of Darwin's *The Origin of Species,* Muller returned to the theme of improving human beings by genetic means. The trilogy of physical, intellectual, and moral characteristics reappeared in Muller's essay, "The Guidance of Human Evolution."[46]

[I]ncreasing attention can be paid to what is called the physical side: bettering the genetic foundations of health, vigor, and longevity; reducing the need for sleep; bringing the induction of sedation and stimulation under better voluntary control; and increasing physical tolerances and aptitudes in general.[47]

• • •

But at least so far as intelligence is concerned, there are no indications that we are now approaching any physiologically set limit or optimum. It is quite evident that we could benefit indefinitely by a continued increase in our mental powers: to enable us to analyze more profoundly; to recognize more readily common features when they lie deeply buried; to grasp more and more elements of a situation at once and co-ordinately; to see more steps ahead; to think more multidimensionally; and to imagine more creatively.[48]

• • •

Surely in this society most of us could do better if, by nature as well as by training, we had less tendency to quick anger, blinding fear, strong jealousy, and self-deceiving egotism. At the same time we need a strengthening and extension of the tendencies toward kindliness, affection, and fellow feeling in general, especially toward those personally far removed from us. These impulses should become sufficiently dynamic to issue in helpful action. As regards other affective traits, there is much room for broadening and deepening our capacity to appreciate both natural and man-made constructions, to interpret with fuller empathy the expressions of others, to create ever richer combinations of our own impressions, and to communicate them to others more adequately.[49]

In the following sections we accept the three-part framework developed by Muller as a helpful categorization of possible human enhancements.[50] We note in passing that Muller seems to have identified artistic imagination with his second category, the intellectual qualities, and that certain affective characteristics and communication skills were associated with the third category, the moral qualities of human beings.

Physical Enhancements

We begin with the question of physical enhancements because such enhancements may seem to be less threatening to the essence or central core of a human being, or to human nature in general, than changes in the intellectual or moral spheres. In our discussion, a further distinction may become quite important, namely, the distinction between health-related physical enhancements and non–health-related physical enhancements. This distinction roughly parallels the distinction between surgery for the treatment or prevention of disease and cosmetic surgery.

Health-related enhancements. Are there health-related physical enhancements that do not involve genetic intervention but that we currently consider to be ethically acceptable? In current medical practice, the best example of a widely accepted health-related physical enhancement is *immunization against infectious diseases*. With immunizations against diseases like polio and hepatitis B, what we are saying is, in effect, "The immune system that we inherited from our parents may not be adequate to ward off certain viruses if we are exposed to them. Therefore, we will enhance the capabilities of our immune system by priming it to fight against these viruses."[51]

From the current practice of immunization against particular diseases, it would seem to be only a small step to try to enhance the general functioning of the immune system by genetic means. Suppose, for example, that a means were discovered for preserving the youth and vigor of the immune system without causing the system to overreact and to attack the individual's own cells or tissues. One of the positive results of such an immune-system enhancement might be that our bodies would be more successful in identifying and attacking cancer cells as we age. This improvement, in turn, might reduce the incidence of breast cancer and prostate cancer in older women and men. Similarly, older people with genetically enhanced immune systems might be better able to ward off potentially life-threatening infectious diseases like influenza and pneumonia.

We should acknowledge that there are some potential technical problems with the proposal to provide a *general* enhancement of human immune-system function. The immune system is always in a very delicate balance: it must be vigilant in its surveillance of foreign threats to the body, but at the same time it must not be so vigorous that it attacks the body's own cells. In other words, hypersensitization of the immune system would not contribute to physical health; it could, in fact, lead to auto-immune disease. The key notion here is to achieve a rejuvenation of the immune system, so that it recovers its earlier alertness and vigor, or better still, a preventive intervention that keeps the immune system young as the human organism advances through middle age to the later years.

In our view, the genetic enhancement of immune-system function would be morally justifiable if this kind of enhancement assisted in preventing disease and did not cause offsetting harms to the people treated by the technique. This general conclusion would not, of course, answer a series of other questions that surely would arise. For example, should gene-mediated immune-system enhancement be employed only with consenting adults, or would parents be morally permitted to accept the enhancement on behalf of their children? Should this important enhancement be made available to everyone or only to those who could pay for it? Would a germ-line approach to this enhancement be ethically acceptable? And should this kind of enhancement be made a mandatory part of public-health programs, as childhood immunizations often are? All of these questions parallel issues that have been discussed in the preceding two chapters.

Non-health-related enhancements. A second kind of potential genetic enhancement would be non–health-related. Here we have in mind enhancements like a more muscular physique, greater energy and endurance, or wrinkle-free skin. These kinds of enhancements are reminiscent of attempts by athletes to gain a competitive edge, of parental efforts to use growth hormone for children of low-normal stature, and of cosmetic surgery. The major difference between current efforts to achieve enhancement and the kind of enhancement being discussed here is that we are here considering gene-mediated enhancements, the effects of which could be permanent for an individual (with somatic cell enhancement) and the effects of which could be transmitted to an individual's descendants (with germ-line enhancement).[52]

In our analysis of the morality of such non-health-related genetic enhancement proposals, we need to draw at least three kinds of distinctions. First, genetic enhancements that are freely chosen by consenting adults can be distinguished from enhancements that might be chosen by parents on behalf of their young children. Second, genetic enhancements that affect competition in sports can be distinguished from those that do not. And third, somatic cell enhancements can be distinguished from germ-line enhancements. In the case of each of these distinctions, one member of the pair is more difficult to justify than the other.

If a consenting adult chooses to undergo cosmetic surgery to change the shape of his or her larger-than-average nose, other persons generally do not have strong grounds for moral objection unless they are asked to help pay for this elective surgery or unless such surgery causes a shortage of surgeons for more urgent life-saving care. However, a parent's desire to employ cosmetic surgery to revise the shape of a child's larger-than-average nose would probably be questioned by the child's pediatrician, as well as by any surgeon asked to perform the operation.[53] In a similar way, there might relatively little moral objection to an adult's attempting to employ gene-mediated growth-hormone treatment in the attempt to add muscle to his or her frame. (Similar stipulations would need to apply, namely, that other people should not be asked to pay for this intervention as a "medical" treatment and that this gene-mediated enhancement should not divert health personnel or growth-hormone treatment from those whose need for it can be defined as "medical.") However, a parental attempt to employ genetic techniques to add muscle bulk to an 8-year-old, for the sake of the child's appearance alone, would surely encounter resistance from the child's pediatrician and perhaps conscientious objection by the professional(s) invited to perform the enhancement.

The context of sports also adds an important dimension to discussions of non-health-related genetic enhancements. Here the most famous sports cases from the past have involved steroid use by sprinters and weight lifters and blood doping by participants in long-distance cycling events. The primary concern regarding the use of such substances or procedures is that they may give users a competitive advantage that at least seems to be unfair. For example, the desire to promote fairness in Olympic competition has given rise to an elaborate system of testing athletes for the use of banned substances.[54] In a parallel way, the use of gene-mediated enhancement by a few athletes would raise concerns about unfair advantage or a nonlevel playing field. The question would surely arise as to whether the athletes should be divided into two categories—those who had received genetic enhancement and those who had not. Further, unless and until the vectors employed in genetic intervention are much more precise and efficient than the vectors of the early 1990s, there will remain at least a theoretical concern about harming some of the treated cells. In the context of life-threatening disease these theoretical risks can be outweighed by potential health benefits. In the context of performance enhancement in sports or standardized testing, the projected benefit may not outweigh the potential harm.[55]

The third important distinction is between somatic cell and germ-line enhancements that are non-health-related. As we noted above, there is less ethical concern about decisions that adults make on their own behalf than about proxy decisions made on behalf of their children. This concern would be magnified if enhancement decisions affected not only the next generation (with a somatic cell enhancement in a child) but also that child's own children and grandchildren and so on. In this case an enhancement would be chosen in order to provide some kind of perceived advantage—in musculature, in performance, in appearance, or in some other non–health-related sphere—to *all* of one's descendants. It is, of course, true that the descendants could elect to reverse the enhancement that their forebears had bequeathed to them, but they would have to take action, by undergoing a kind of genetic procedure, in order to do so. If the descendants also wished to prevent their children and grandchildren from inheriting the enhancement, their task of genetic intervention would be even more formidable.

We are not prepared at this point in the chapter to condemn all such efforts at germ-line enhancement for non-health-related reasons. Rather, we wish to note that the number of future persons directly affected by a decision could be very large and that the indirect effects on third parties of such a decision by one couple could be exceedingly great. Further, one would want to examine the effects of a system in which various couples were competing to give their descendants significant physical advantages in the struggle for success. We will return to these questions after examining the three general types of enhancements.

A dubious case: size. A first example of a genetic enhancement that is not health-related would be gene-mediated growth-hormone treatment for children who are likely to be short-statured as adults. Human growth hormone produced by recombinant DNA methods is currently used in approximately 20,000 children in the United States.[56] About 75% of the children under treatment are growth-hormone deficient. In these children, growth hormone seems to stimulate growth, strengthen bones, and build muscle mass. Most of the remaining 25% are girls who have a chromosomal abnormality called Turner syndrome. Although girls with this condition secrete normal amounts of growth hormone, their final height averages 4 feet, 8 inches. Clinical studies of whether growth-hormone treatment increases the height of girls who have Turner syndrome are in progress.[57] Some children who are short because their parents are short, but who are not growth-hormone deficient, are also receiving growth hormone, but it is not yet clear whether this intervention simply speeds up the start of growth or also affects final height. The cost of treating children with synthetic human growth hormone is considerable, averaging between $10,000 and $30,000 per year in the United States.[58]

In our view, gene-mediated growth-hormone treatment for children who have a growth-hormone deficiency would be a health-related enhancement because of the multiple beneficial effects of the treatment in the bodies of children. However, it is much more difficult to justify the use of this genetic intervention for short-statured children who are not growth-hormone deficient. Our reason for asserting this difference is that short-statured people are often physically healthy in every aspect of their physiological functioning. An alternative to genetic enhancement in their case would be to attempt to change social attitudes toward short-statured people. This kind of change in social attitudes would not suffice for children who have growth-hormone deficiency.

Clearly one's notions of health and disease enter into judgments of this sort. We are attempting to draw a sharp line between bona fide illness, on the one hand, and physical traits that can lead to discouragement or discrimination or both, on the other. In our view, genetic "enhancements" that would alter stature or skin color or gender fall into this second category rather than qualifying as health-related.

A difficult case: the need for sleep. Suppose that there were a gene-mediated enhancement technique that reduced one's daily need for sleep by 50%, with no loss of attentiveness during the waking hours. Would this enhancement be health-related or not? And, on balance, would such an enhancement be morally justifiable? (Note that we are not espousing the more radical proposal that the need for sleep be totally abolished. We propose a reduction rather than abolition in part because of concerns about the possible need for dreaming and other types of brain activity during sleep and also because of the close correlation between sexual activity and sleep.)[59]

We raise the issue of sleep because there seems to be something inherently odd about our spending, on average, between one-fourth and one-third of our lives in a state of unconsciousness. It is true that all nonhuman animals sleep. Further, we often feel refreshed and better able to go about our daily activities after a period of sleep. But would human beings have to be designed in this way? Could we not develop technical means for enabling our bodies to rest even as we are active?

Some preliminary analysis may help here. Most of us know people who seem to be able to get along on very little sleep—perhaps only 4 or 5 hours per night. While such people may fall outside the normal range, statistically speaking, there is nothing unnatural or morally objectionable in their daily schedules merely because they need less sleep than the average person. We are also aware that at least for short periods of time we can get by with less than the usual amount of sleep—for example, when a term paper is due, or a grant application must be completed, or a move to a new home occurs. We may even use nongenetic means to assist us to stay awake during such periods; coffee, NoDoz pills, or even more powerful stimulants may be the drugs of choice. But after such an intense period of sustained effort and reduced sleep, we may find that we need to "crash," to take time off from daily activities for extra rest and perhaps compensatory sleep. In these deadline situations followed by a catch-up phase, it almost seems as if we borrow waking time from the future, only to have to pay off the loan within the next few days or weeks.

We acknowledge that there may be limits set by human physiology *as it currently exists* that will make a reduction in the need for sleep technically infeasible. For example, if there is for each person an approximate biological limit on the number of waking hours in a lifetime, then a genetic enhancement leading to a reduced need for sleep would simply compress an individual's lifetime into fewer years. The total number of waking hours would remain the same. It is possible that, given the choice, some individuals would prefer to "budget" their years of life in a way that involved a smaller proportion of time spent in sleep, even if a side effect of this enhancement were that they would die at a younger age than they otherwise would have. For example, graduate or professional students might prefer to complete their degree programs earlier rather than later. Or the chief executive of a small business might prefer to get his or her company off to a running start. However, if the effect of such an accelerated investment of waking hours were in fact a shortening of one's life, then a reduction by genetic means in the need for sleep might be perceived as a tradeoff rather than a genuine enhancement.

In our view, it is difficult to condemn in advance and in principle genetic intervention aimed at reducing people's need for sleep. Regardless of whether the waking hours are merely shifted forward in a shortened life-span or actually added to the expected quota of waking hours in a lifetime, some people might be able to provide good reasons for choosing this enhancement. However, again in this case the potential social effects of such choices would need to be carefully assessed. Further, the question of access to this enhancement or its allocation within society would surely need to be addressed.

An even more difficult case: aging. In this final scenario of physical enhancement we hypothesize that a genetic intervention might be able to add years of
healthy, vigorous life to the normal life-span. Would such an enhancement be
regarded as health-related because it delays the physical decline associated with
aging? And would such an enhancement be morally justifiable, without regard to
its being categorized as health-related or non-health-related?

The physiological assumption underlying this anti-aging proposal is that human
cells—and perhaps all cells—are genetically programmed to be able to divide only
a certain number of times.[60] When a sufficient proportion of our cells reach this
inherent biological limit, the organism as a whole manifests signs of aging, and
then dies. In human beings this biological limit can be seen most clearly in el-
derly people who do not die because of cancer or heart disease but simply because their bodies seem to wear out. In 20th-century human beings this built-in
limit of a *natural life-span* seems to be set at approximately 100–120 years.

Perhaps the most important question to be asked about the proposal to extend
the duration of healthy life by genetic means is: why undertake such an effort at
all? Various answers to this question can be given. One answer would appeal to
the goals of medicine, among which are the goals of promoting health and
extending life. Another answer might be: to preserve our relationships with
people whom we admire and respect. One thinks, for example, of children who
never learn to know their grandparents or who know them for only a short time.
Other candidates for genetic life extension might be great artists, gifted musicians, and esteemed political leaders. A third possible answer to the "why" question is: "We find life, on balance, to be enjoyable, and we would like to continue in the enjoyment of life as long as possible." Or, one might accent the rapid
technological change that occurs within the span of a current human life and
simply be curious to know what additional changes will occur within the succeeding decades.

The precise shape of the genetic-life-extension question depends in part on the
number of years of additional life envisioned. Fifty additional years might appear
to be manageable within current institutional arrangements. A doubling of the
normal life-span, to 200–240 years, would probably lead to significant social
adjustments. And a normal life-span of 1,000 years is difficult to imagine.

Would the extension of life by genetic means be health-related or not? One's
answer to this question depends in part on whether the "normal" aging process is
viewed as a disease. For proponents of natural limits, aging seems to be an
acceptable and indeed essential part of a life trajectory, a fitting conclusion to a
life that helps to give the entire life its meaning and sense of finitude.[61] On the
other hand, the physical decline and even disintegration that overtake some eld-
erly people seem at least akin to a disease process, and some proponents of efforts
to extend the years of healthy life see little dignity in the experience of one's bodily
deterioration.[62]

Again in this case we are unwilling to say in advance that a genetic enhancement aimed at extending the life-span should never be undertaken. However, this proposed application of genetic enhancement raises more profound questions regarding social impact than the other enhancements discussed previously. If large numbers of people extended their life spans by genetic means, there would be an immediate impact on population density. Current social policies on whether to limit the number of children per family would need to be reexamined, as would policies on the normal retirement age. Clearly, the actuaries for the Social Security Trust Fund would need to make new projections in light of the changed situation!

Thus, we neither recommend nor condemn the use of genetic intervention to extend the human life-span.[63] Rather, we merely wish to indicate that genetic techniques may be employed in an effort to push back the last frontiers of human life—aging and death. If these techniques are demonstrated to be safe and efficacious, the proposal to employ them on any significant scale will raise major social policy questions.

Other possible physical enhancements. In an interesting essay entitled "Human Nature Technologically Revisited," H. Tristram Engelhardt, Jr., agrees with Sir Peter Medawar's thesis that "nature does *not* know best" and that genetic evolution is "a story of waste, makeshift, compromise, and blunder."[64] Engelhardt goes on to suggest three physical conditions for which genetic intervention should be considered.

[O]ne can easily develop a short list of human characteristics seriously meriting revision at some time in the future when our capacities with germline genetic engineering are fully matured. These would include (1) presbyopia, the nearly universal difficulty experienced by humans over 40 in achieving a short focal length, as needed for reading; (2) menopause, with its concomitant osteoporosis (and the sequelae of collapsed vertebrae, broken hips, etc.) and senile vaginitis;[a] and (3) the shortened life expectancy of males (in 1985 males in the United States had a life expectancy of 71.2 years, as opposed to 78.2 years for women), which is in part due to genetically determined increased risks of diseases—such as myocardial infarction and cancer of the prostate.[65]

For Peter Medawar "aberrations" and "miscarriages" of the immunological process are some of the most important flaws resulting from the human evolutionary process. The consequences are, in Medawar's words, "[a]naphylactic shock, allergy, and hypersensitivity."[66]

We will not examine in detail the physical conditions suggested by Engelhardt and Medawar as candidates for future genetic enhancement. We do note, however, that each of these physiological processes is an aspect of species-typical functioning for human beings in the twentieth century. Thus, any effort to modify these physiological processes and their resulting conditions will be an attempt to go beyond species-typical functioning toward an ideal of better-than-typical physical functioning.

Transition to the Question of Intellectual and Moral Enhancements

We turn now from the relatively straightforward arena of physical enhancements to what some commentators have called "the genetic basis of complex human behaviors."[67] These behaviors are studied by researchers in a lively and diverse academic field called *behavioral genetics*. Research in behavioral genetics relies on a variety of methods. In the 1960s through the 1980s, the principal approach was to study extended families, adopted children, and identical (*monozygotic*) and fraternal (*dizygotic*) twins for clues to the heritability of behavioral traits. In the 1990s this traditional method was joined by the new power of molecular genetics. Sometimes a single gene or a small group of genes is identified and connected to a human behavioral trait or disorder. The discovery of the fragile-X syndrome and its connection to mental retardation illustrates this approach. In other cases, molecular geneticists study populations to derive clues to the locations of genes that may be associated with human behavior or disease. Geneticists call this search the effort to discover *quantitative trait loci (QTL)*.[68] These loci are neither necessary nor sufficient for the development of a particular disease or trait. Rather, they seem to denote multiple genes that have effects of varying sizes. QTL can be thought of as indicators of susceptibility or a predisposition to a certain outcome. A recent finding based on use of the QTL method was that a gene connected to heart disease, the *Apo-E* gene, is associated with a dramatically increased risk of developing late-onset Alzheimer disease.[69]

The intellectual roots of behavioral genetics reach back at least into the 19th century and especially to the writings of two English scholars, Charles Darwin and his half-cousin Francis Galton. In his book, *The Descent of Man*, Darwin wrote:

I have elsewhere[a] so fully discussed the subject of Inheritance, that I need here add hardly anything. A greater number of facts have been collected with respect to the transmission of the most trifling, as well as of the most important characters in man, than in any of the lower animals; though the facts are copious enough with respect to the latter. So in regard to mental qualities, their transmission is manifest in our dogs, horses, and other domestic animals. Besides special tastes and habits, general intelligence, courage, bad and good temper, &c., are certainly transmitted. With man we see similar facts in almost every family; and we know now, through the admirable labours of Mr. Galton,[b] that genius which implies a wonderfully complex combination of high faculties, tends to be inherited; and, on the other hand, it is too certain that insanity and deteriorated mental powers likewise run in families.[70]

In his earlier book, *On the Origin of Species*, Darwin had discussed the inheritance of behavioral traits in his chapter on instinct (Chapter VII). After noting the difference between animal instincts that had developed in the state of nature and instincts that had developed during domestication, Darwin described striking behavioral traits of one domesticated species, the dog.

But let us look to the familiar case of several breeds of dogs: it cannot be doubted that young pointers (I have myself seen a striking instance) will sometimes point and even back other dogs the very first time that they are taken out; retrieving is certainly in some degree inherited by retrievers; and a tendency to run round, instead of at, a flock of sheep, by shepherd-dogs. I cannot see that these actions, performed without experience by the young, and in nearly the same manner by each individual, performed with eager delight by each breed, and without the end being known,—for the young pointer can no more know that he points to aid his master, than the white butterfly knows why she lays her eggs on the leaf of the cabbage,—I cannot see that these actions differ essentially from true [that is, natural] instincts.[71]

Had Darwin been writing in the era after the rediscovery of Gregor Mendel's work (published in 1866 but not widely known until 1900), he would surely have tied his discussion of instincts to genes.

During the 20th century the scientific findings of Darwin, Galton, and later researchers concerning the inheritance of behavioral traits have been employed for both destructive and constructive purposes. One of the saddest chapters in the history of this century has been the misuse of such findings, with a large admixture of pseudoscience, to support racist, xenophobic, coercive, and brutal eugenics programs. In fact, the programs of involuntary sterilization in the United States and of sterilization and extermination in Nazi Germany so traumatized the academic community in the United States and continental Europe that discussion of inherited behavioral traits was virtually a taboo topic between 1940 and 1960.[72] A new stage of academic discussion was signaled in 1960 by the publication of John L. Fuller and William R. Thompson's book, *Behavior Genetics*.[73] This thoroughly documented work considered five major topics in human behavioral genetics: "variation in sensory and perceptual processes," "response processes," "intellectual abilities," "personality and temperament," and "mental disorders."[74] From the inception of the field of behavioral genetics, most of its practitioners have consciously sought to avoid the racist and discriminatory overtones that accompanied the earlier eugenics movement.

We should note that behavioral genetics as a field has been accused by some critics of going too far in ascribing behavior to genetic, as distinct from social and cultural, factors. For example, a recent review of the field in *Scientific American* was entitled, "Trends in Behavioral Genetics: Eugenics Revisited."[75] In contrast, a mediating position is adopted by Paul Billings, Jonathan Beckwith, and Joseph Alper, who draw a sharp distinction between molecular and nonmolecular (social-scientific) genetic studies of human behavior. In their view, molecular genetic correlations discovered through DNA-based linage studies and the biochemical analysis of genes are much more reliable, and much easier to confirm, than, for example, twin studies that attempt to distinguish between environmental and genetic factors in behavior.[76] Robert Plomin, a leading scholar in behavioral genetics, also adopts a mediating view. While asserting that "genetic factors play a major role in behavioural dimensions and disorders," he also concedes that "In the United States especially, the pendulum of scientific fashion seems to be swinging too far from environmentalism towards a genetic determinism."[77]

In the next two sections of this chapter we will explore several of the themes that have been central to the renewed interest in behavioral genetics in the 1990s.[78] These include cognitive ability and disability, personality traits, sexual orientation, addictive behavior, psychiatric disorders, and aggression. As we address each topic, we will attempt to remind ourselves and our readers that in almost every case we are considering genetic factors or influences in human behavior, rather than genetic *determinants* of such behavior. Environmental factors and the intentions of persons are also important components in any comprehensive analysis of human action.[79]

Intellectual Enhancements

The phrase "intellectual enhancements" might seem to connote, first and foremost, attempts to raise the intelligence level of the recipients of the genetic intervention. Thus, in a questionnaire employed by the Louis Harris organization in national surveys taken in 1986 and again in 1992, respondents were asked whether they would approve of "scientists changing the makeup of human cells" in order to "improve the intelligence that children would inherit."[80] However, neuroscientists have discovered that the human brain is multifaceted and that the various functions of the brain can be carried on in at least partial independence of one another.[81] It may therefore be useful to begin the discussion of possible intellectual enhancements by considering a less ambitious project than improving the amorphous set of characteristics called "intelligence."

Memory. A relatively modest intellectual enhancement effort would be the attempt to increase the efficiency of long-term memory. To make this example more concrete, let us consider the possibility of doubling the efficiency of long-term memory by genetic means. Such a genetic intervention would not mean that the recipient would remember everything that he or she heard or read or saw. Rather, it would mean that the person with enhanced memory efficiency would be more like the few people with photographic memories than before the intervention. In other words, if the average person usually retains about 20% of what he or she hears, reads, or sees,[82] that figure would rise to 40% if the intervention were successful.

In academic settings memory enhancement would seem, at first blush, to be a highly desirable kind of genetic intervention. Teachers would be able to prepare for classes and write articles and books more efficiently because they would have more information at their fingertips. Similarly, insofar as test-taking and paper-writing by students call upon the remembrance of important facts and concepts, these important student activities would also be facilitated by memory enhancement. In nonacademic settings, as well, there would be a useful role for memory enhancement. Think, for example, of a travel agent remembering the names of clients or beautiful destinations for family vacations. Alternatively, think of an attorney remembering more of the facts of the case or more of the arguments put forward by the opposing side.

What are the major arguments against memory enhancement by means of genetic intervention? One kind of objection is purely technical, and technical information will be needed to determine whether or not it represents a serious obstacle to memory enhancement. The objection is that the human brain has a finite capacity, and that when that upper limit is reached, new information must displace old information. Thus, beyond a certain point, memory enhancement might not represent a net benefit. Perhaps the closest analogies for thinking about this possibility come from the microcomputer world. Every microcomputer has a certain amount of random access memory (or RAM). When one or more programs exceed the capacity of the computer's RAM, the program(s) cannot run. One can also think of this first objection in terms of the storage devices for microcomputers. If a new document or program requires more storage space than the remaining open space on a diskette or a hard disk, old information will have to be deleted to create space for "saving" new information.

If the limits on storage capacity in the long-term memory are, in fact, an obstacle to memory enhancement as outlined above, the question of memory enhancement may, in fact, take on a new shape. Rather than facilitating the encoding and decoding of information into a huge memory facility with large amounts of unused space, the genetic intervention may have to create more storage space as well as make our use of the space more efficient. In other words, the number of memory chips in the computer may have to be increased or a second hard disk may have to be added to the system.

The nontechnical objection to memory enhancement usually takes the following form: "We all have very unpleasant and even traumatic experiences. It is therefore a great benefit to be able to forget." Proponents of memory enhancement can respond to this objection as follows. "Selective forgetting is a very important mechanism for coping with negative or traumatic memories. However, we assume that the same filtering system that allows humans to remember selectively now would also continue to operate in the brains of people who have undergone genetic memory enhancement. Preclinical studies in laboratory animals will be helpful in establishing this assumption."

Until now, we have been considering the enhancement of memory that falls within the normal range. However, there is in human beings a specific condition of declining memory efficiency that is associated with aging, namely, *senile dementia* in its various forms. Although senile dementia in a certain fraction of the aging population represents species-typical functioning, we have no hesitation in calling such dementia a disease within the medical model. As noted above, two kinds of dementia of the Alzheimer type have been linked with genetic loci—one with two chromosomes, the other with a specific gene. Current studies of drugs and hormones will perhaps one day be supplemented by genetic approaches to the treatment and even the prevention of senile dementia.[83]

General cognitive ability. A second potential target of genetic enhancement is "intelligence," or, more modestly, the kind of general cognitive ability that can be measured by standardized tests like the Wechsler Intelligence Scale, as well as by newer tests that attempt to analyze how the brain processes various kinds of information.[84] There is, of course, considerable controversy surrounding the question of whether general cognitive ability is, at least in part, an inherited trait. The best available evidence suggests that, in preadolescent children, approximately 40–50% of general cognitive ability is closely correlated with inheritance.[85] A recent study of 332 monozygotic and 242 dizygotic twin pairs aged 7–16 estimated the heritability of verbal comprehension at 0.44, of perceptual organization at 0.50, and of freedom from distractibility at 0.49.[86] Shared and nonshared environmental influences accounted for the remaining differences between the two kinds of twins.

One possible condition for which the enhancement of general cognitive ability might be considered is fragile-X syndrome, the most common genetic cause of mental retardation. This disorder affects one in 1,250 males in the United States. The molecular basis of fragile-X is now known to be a triplet (CGG) repeat in a region of the *FMR-1* gene on the X chromosome. Tragically, the number of triplet repeats increases with each succeeding generation, and the number of repeats is correlated with the age of onset and the severity of the disorder. Fifty copies of the CGG repeat is the usual number. Any number of repeats above 200 compromises cognitive functioning. A few hundred repeats may cause only a learning disability with normal intelligence, while thousands of repeats cause severe mental retardation.[87] A genetic intervention that removed excess repeats or counteracted their influence would clearly fall into the category of treating or preventing a disorder that would otherwise make it impossible for a person to enjoy species-typical cognitive functioning.

Again in this case a conceptual question arises: Is the use of genetic intervention to raise a person's level of cognitive functioning to (or at least near) the mean really "enhancement" or would it be more appropriately called "remediation"? If this kind of intervention is viewed as remediation, it closely parallels the role of therapy in the treatment of disease. In other words, the line between the upper and lower boxes in our two-by-two matrix (see page xvii) may not always be sharp and clear.

But what can be said about hypothetical efforts to employ genetic intervention to improve the cognitive functioning of people who are already within the normal range? Among philosophers and theologians, it is the British philosopher Jonathan Glover who has argued most extensively and most passionately for the desirability of "transcending intellectual limitations." In his book *What Sort of People Should There Be?* Glover writes:

A possible role for positive genetic engineering would be to raise our intellectual capacity. One day, perhaps remote from now, we may start to feel that we are coming up against the in-built limitations of our ability to understand the universe.

• • •

[O]ur unmodified intellectual equipment [might be inadequate for] extending our scientific understanding of the world. Just as calculus is too much for a dog's brain to grasp, so some parts of physics might turn out to be too difficult for us as we are. No doubt it would be hard to be sure that we were pressing against our limitations. But, faced with a continuing lack of progress on very baffling problems, we might come to suspect this. And we might have some thoughts on what changes in brain functioning could make a difference.

• • •

Any programme of genetic engineering to modify our intellectual functioning would obviously have to be very cautious and experimental. But, once it showed signs of working without bad side-effects, it seems likely that some parents would choose to have children who would transcend our traditional limitation. Because our growing understanding of the world is so central a part of why it is good to be human, it would be very tempting for us to break through our genetic intellectual limitations.

If we do have such limits, and do decide to transcend them, our descendants may be glad. To them, our decision might mean escape from a kind of claustrophobia. For the alternative would be to have an understanding of the world that was incomplete yet permanently static. And this kind of stifling is something the human race has not known since we first woke up and started to ask our questions.[88]

Glover is clearly concerned with improving the cognitive ability of people whose intellectual powers already lie comfortably within the normal range. Although this question is often raised by parents on behalf of their minor children, it can also be asked by an adult considering whether to undergo an intervention for the enhancement of his or her own cognitive ability. The issue of somatic-cell germ-line intervention is also important in this case. Somatic cell enhancements of cognitive ability, whether performed in children or adults, would not be passed on to future generations.

What gives many people pause, as they consider the genetic enhancement of cognitive ability, is the specter of overly zealous parents pushing such a technology to extremes with their own children.[89] In a society with fierce competition for entry into the best nursery schools, with a strong emphasis on success in Little League baseball and high-school basketball, with the introduction of children to computers at ever-younger ages, is it likely that parents would exercise moderation in their use of genetic means to improve cognitive ability? For example, would the parents of a child with a measured I.Q. of 125 be inclined to tack on an extra 15–20 points, just as insurance? Lying just below the surface in these questions are questions about socioeconomic status and about whether our long-term goal as a society is to move toward greater equality or toward more pronounced differences between the haves and the have-nots.

At the same time, however, it is difficult to condemn all efforts by people whose cognitive ability falls within the normal range to enhance that ability by genetic means. Adults who decided to improve their own intellectual functioning by somatic cell intervention would probably be able to cite multiple plausible reasons for wanting to undertake such an intervention. Thus, in our view, the presumption should be in favor of their freedom to elect this enhancement, unless and until the practice of enhancement presents a clear and present danger to society. In contrast, children would probably need to be protected against one additional form of potential abuse by adults, including well-meaning parents. At the same time, however, scope should be allowed for the legitimate exercise of parental and familial autonomy.[90] Germ-line enhancement of cognitive abilities would affect multiple generations of descendants, but they could presumably reverse the enhancement if they perceived it to be detrimental to them. Perhaps most difficult to resolve would be the distribution questions that would surround this powerful new technology. We will return to these questions later in this chapter.

Moral Enhancements

The third category of possible improvements in the human species suggested by H.J. Muller and the cosigners of the "Geneticists' Manifesto" might best be called *moral enhancements*. We acknowledge that this topic is the most controversial that we will discuss in this book. The topic easily conjures up images of mind control (à la *Brave New World* or *A Clockwork Orange*). It is perhaps even feared that moral enhancements would signal the end of morality as we know it.

There will surely be formidable technical obstacles to the genetic enhancement of moral characteristics. Such characteristics are intimately related to the personality of an individual. Moral traits are clearly related to many genes, perhaps even many hundreds of genes. In addition, the early training of each individual and each individual's social environment interact with what in most cases seem to be, at most, genetic predispositions to antisocial behavior.[91]

The clearest case of a close correlation between a gene and impulsive, antisocial behavior involves males from a large extended family in the Netherlands. According to the human geneticists who studied eight affected males from this family,

Behavioral problems were reported for all eight affected males. Abnormal behavior was documented for affected males in at least four different sibships living in different parts of the country at different times. Most striking were repeated episodes of aggressive, sometimes violent, behavior, occurring in all eight affected males. Aggressive behavior was usually triggered by anger and was often out of proportion to the provocation. Aggressive behavior tended to cluster in periods of 1–3 d[ays], during which the affected male would sleep very little and would experience frequent night terrors. . . . In one instance, an affected male was convicted of the rape of his sister, at 23 years. He was transferred to an institution for psychopaths, where he was described as quiet and easy to handle. In spite of this, fights occurred with other inmates, and he was repeatedly transferred to a different pavilion. At the age of 35 years, while working in the fields, he stabbed one of the wardens in the chest with a pitchfork, after having been told to get on with his work. Another affected male tried to run over his boss with a car at the sheltered workshop where he was employed, after having been told that his work was not up to par. A third affected male would enter his sisters' bedrooms at night, armed with a knife, and force them to undress. At least two affected males in this family are known arsonists. This latter behavior appears linked to stressful circumstances, such as the death of a relative.[92]

Through linkage analysis the researchers studying this family were able to determine that a mutation in the gene that produces the enzyme monoamine oxidase A was present on the X chromosome in all five of the affected males who were available for direct study. Biochemical analysis of 24-hour urine samples from three of these affected males revealed abnormal levels of the neurotransmitters serotonin and norepinephrine.[93] In both animal and human studies, high levels of norepinephrine and low levels of serotonin have been associated with increased aggression.[94]

If the results of the Dutch study are replicated in other studies, a genetic marker will be available for diagnosing a rare genetic condition that is closely correlated with impulsive, violent behavior. In the future, it seems likely that additional genetic markers associated with impulsive, aggressive, or violent behavior will be discovered. We base this assertion on several observations. First, as Darwin had already noted in the 19th century, the success of animal breeders in domesticating dogs, cats, horses, and other species suggests that traits of relative tameness can be identified and selected for. More recently, through repeated selection researchers have succeeded in breeding both high- and low-aggressive populations of mice and foxes from single gene pools.[95] Second, correlations between the levels of specific hormones (for example, testosterone) and neurotransmitters (for example, dopamine) and aggressive behavior have been postulated. At present we see no clear evidence for a definite effect of any of these hormones or neurotransmitters on behavior. However, if definite effects are found in the future, they may in turn be traced to genetic factors.[96] Third, behavioral geneticists who have studied large cohorts of identical and fraternal twins have concluded that the genetic component of variation in five major personality traits which they call the *super factors* is approximately 40%.[97] One end of the spectrum for the trait of *agreeableness* includes the descriptors "quarrelsome," "aggressive," and "vindictive." Similarly, the personality measures for the trait of *conscientiousness* find that some humans are "impulsive, careless, irresponsible."[98] Both of these personality factors, while not simply equivalent to moral traits, are closely related to individual moral character and are likely to give rise to actions that are at best indifferent to the welfare of others and at worst clearly antisocial.

Several caveats need to be entered at this point. First, we are not anticipating the discovery of crime genes or violence genes through further research. Rather, we expect that, in most cases at least, multiple genes will interact in complicated ways to produce a higher-than-average predisposition to violent or antisocial behavior. In other words, we agree with the general point made by Robert Plomin when he writes:

For complex behaviors, the problem is that few candidate genes are known that are as specific as the apolipoprotein genes associated with cardiovascular disease. Nonetheless, many genes expressed in the brain are likely to make very small contributions to the genetic variance for complex behaviors, which can be detected with large samples.[99]

Second, some types of "aggressive" and "quarrelsome" behavior are either morally neutral or even morally laudable. When aggression is channeled into academic or athletic competition, within reasonable bounds, it can contribute in important ways to an individual's self-development. Further, there are some situations for which quarrelsome behavior seems the appropriate response. One thinks, for example, of religious figures like the Hebrew prophets and Jesus or of 20th-century figures like Mohandas K. Gandhi and Martin Luther King. To their contemporary opponents, these people must have seemed to be querulous trouble-makers, yet many of us applaud the efforts of these historical figures to combat hypocrisy and injustice.

There are, however, some kinds of disregard for other people and some kinds of aggression against other people that clearly merit moral disapproval. We are thinking, in particular, of two kinds of disregard and aggression for which genetic intervention may be considered as at least one component of an overall response. The first kind of disregard and aggression could be characterized as clearly anti-social or sociopathic behavior by certain people within a society. In this case, the goal of the intervention would be to move behavior that is outside the range of species-typical human functioning to some point within the normal range. This kind of intervention would again look like remediation and would be at least *akin to* therapy for disease. The second kind of disregard and aggression is the kind that characterizes most human beings, at least in our dispositions and often in our overt actions or failures to act. In this case, the goal of the intervention would be to move species-typical functioning itself toward a more conscientious and agreeable norm.

In a 1990 essay, H. Tristram Engelhardt, Jr., provides an interesting example of the first kind of moral enhancement. Engelhardt envisions a time when "wide-ranging genetic germline engineering becomes possible" and asserts that at such a time "the challenge of the governance of a polity will need to be restated."[100] Engelhardt continues:

It may indeed turn out that there is a range of human antisocial dispositions and inclinations that can be more easily modified through genetic engineering than through education or through coercive or instructive social structures. One will then need to ask what balance among the influences of social structures, education, and biological structures a community should find endorsable as means for ensuring the existence of a peaceable community. For the purpose of example and discussion, one might agree with the argument of some sociobiologists who have contended that the inclination of young males to kill other young males is biologically based and was established because of its contribution to inclusive fitness.[a] In contemporary environments, when young male belligerence is augmented not only by firearms but by nuclear weapons, their contribution to inclusive fitness may have been altered.[b] Should such problems be addressed only through education and the law (or other social structures), were a simple genetic solution more effective? Indeed, if it is determined that some syndromes of marked lack of impulse control and of violence have a significant genetic component,[c] it will likely be the case that many would-be parents will want their progeny "treated" because of both familial and social concerns.[101]

Disregard for others and aggression toward others is also part of the general human condition. Some of the most eloquent passages in Jonathan Glover's book *What Sort of People Should There Be?* are those in which he describes the "emotional and imaginative limitations" of human beings.

In optimistic moments, we may hope that our history of cruelty and killing is part of a primitive past, to be left behind as civilization develops. But the events of our own century do not suggest that this process has gone far. We still know large-scale killing, sometime of the inhabitants of entire cities in war, sometime extermination of whole peoples as a deliberate policy. We are familiar with the effects of napalm, and not surprised by the daily use of torture in many parts of the world. Less dramatically, but with similar terrible effects, we are used to our own passivity in the face of so much hunger, disease and poverty.

• • •

[It] is hard not to see the limitations of human sympathy, and how easily it can be switched off. We acquiesce in avoidable misery.[102]

Because of his pessimistic reading of human nature, Glover is open to the moral enhancement of human beings by genetic means.[103]

In the remarks that follow we will ask the reader to display the personality trait of openness and to engage in what Samuel Taylor Coleridge called "that willing suspension of disbelief."[104] Let us imagine for a moment that in the year 2110 carefully targeted changes in 100 interrelated genetic sites are demonstrated to increase agreeableness or friendliness and to mute the violently aggressive tendencies often exhibited by the human species. In what contexts, if any, would it be morally justifiable to consider the use of genetic intervention to stimulate friendliness and to suppress violent aggression?

With some trepidation we raise a microquestion and a macroquestion. First, would it be ethically permissible for individuals who are not sociopaths but who wish to be more agreeable to accept gene-mediated friendliness-stimulation for themselves—presumably through a somatic cell intervention? Second, would it be ethically permissible or even desirable for governments to undertake mutually verifiable programs of friendliness-stimulation and violent-aggression suppression within their own societies, with the aim of promoting greater international and domestic cooperation? (We assume that treated individuals would continue to be free to choose their own acts but would be more likely than the average 20th-century human to behave in a friendly manner. In other words, a different mix of predispositions would be present after the genetic intervention. We also assume that political and military leaders as well as average citizens would receive the genetic intervention.)

Even in this thought-experiment we do not propose that the genetic approach to conflict resolution should be the sole approach. In our view, moral enhancement by genetic means would be a useful adjunct to other important programs like social and economic reform and education about ethnic, racial, and national groups that are different from one's own. Early childhood education about non-violent means for resolving conflict is especially important, in our view.

There are several credible objections that can be raised against the moral enhancements outlined above. The first is that the technique, even when chosen by an individual for him- or herself, would interfere with human freedom and, by implication, would undermine the practice of morality. However, as we have indicated above, genetic enhancement as we conceive it would influence but not determine the choices that human beings make. Thus, it would be compatible with respect for autonomy. Further, the voluntary choice of an individual to become more friendly and less violently aggressive would be a free and eminently reasonable decision.

Second, moral enhancement implies dissatisfaction or perhaps even disrespect for human nature as it has evolved through millennia. We acknowledge that we are dissatisfied with what we consider to be violently aggressive characteristics of human beings—characteristics that in all probability have genetic correlates. If moral enhancement rendered these genetic factors less influential in human behavior, we would regard that change as an improvement in human nature. We hasten to add that our goal would not be to achieve perfection in human nature but merely to moderate the influence of the violently aggressive tendencies that are clearly part of human nature as it has been transmitted to us.

A third possible objection has been acknowledged by Jonathan Glover, an advocate of intervention. Glover writes, "The value we place on diversity may conflict with the goal of eliminating the more harmful and dangerous side of our nature."[105] We agree that the widespread use of moral enhancement would make certain violently aggressive character traits and actions less prevalent than they are now, but we would welcome their diminution. There would remain a myriad of human personality traits that are quite diverse. In quantitative terms, even if 100 genetic sites were modified in the effort to stimulate friendliness and suppress aggression, there would be 49,900–99,900 genes that remained unchanged and the corresponding possibility of almost infinite variety in personality traits.

Two other objections are religious in character. The first is that moral enhancement would obviate the need for religion's role in the development of good character. Our reply is that genetic enhancement, as we have described it, would be directed only against a few of the most violently aggressive tendencies in human beings. Even with this aggression suppression and the stimulation of an individual's friendliness, there would be ample opportunity for continuing moral improvement within one's chosen religious tradition and community. The second argument—one that is sometimes employed against germ-line intervention of any kind—is that the proposed intervention is tantamount to playing God. It arrogates to human beings a role that was originally played by God in creation and that should remain God's role alone. Without wishing to discuss the arguments for and against theistic belief, we simply note that our proposal in the thought-experiment is fully compatible with theism. In fact, some theologians have argued that human beings should become co-creators with God by seeking to improve the quality of human life.[106]

The most formidable objections to moral enhancement by genetic means are those raised against the moral enhancement of persons other than oneself, whether they are one's children or fellow members of one's society. As in the case of physical and intellectual enhancements, society would probably need to set limits on parental discretion to prevent child abuse. On the other hand, we agree with Engelhardt that many parents would welcome this new technology and that they should be at liberty to use it in their children within reasonable limits.

More difficult to resolve are the issues surrounding the social use of moral enhancement, particularly in those who express opposition to receiving the intervention. Given the noncoercive approach that we have espoused throughout this book, we cannot justify the mandatory use of *any* genetic intervention, even an intervention aimed at moral enhancement. In any social program of genetically based moral enhancement we would want this intervention to be offered to everyone. No one would be forced to accept the intervention. However, we think that many people, perhaps a majority in most societies where it is available, would accept this new technology. This majority, in turn, would help to create a new ethos that might well attract others who were initially skeptical. At the same time, however, the government of this mixed society would have a clear obligation to protect the (more nearly) peaceable community of those who had accepted moral enhancement from any threatened acts of aggression by those who had refused it.

The Selection and Allocation of Genetic Enhancements

One possible approach to the problem of selecting among possible genetic enhancements is contained in philosopher Robert Nozick's discussion of the "genetic supermarket." Nozick writes,

Many biologists tend to think the problem [of genetically engineering desirable human qualities] is one of *design*, of specifying the best types of persons so that biologists can proceed to produce them. Thus they worry over what sort(s) of person there is to be and who will control this process. They do not tend to think, perhaps because it diminishes the importance of their role, of a system in which they run a "genetic supermarket," meeting the individual specifications (within certain moral limits) of prospective parents. Nor do they think of seeing what limited number of types of persons people's choices would converge upon, if indeed there would be any such convergence. This supermarket system has the great virtue that it involves no centralized decision fixing the future human type(s).[107]

A second answer to the question of selecting genetic enhancements is suggested but rejected by Nozick, namely, a central planning mechanism. In this system the planners would presumably select one or more paradigms of physical, intellectual, and moral excellence and (at least) commend them to the population at large. There are at least hints of this approach in geneticist H.J. Muller's 1935 book, *Out of the Night*. Muller proposed attempting to move human evolution toward the personal qualities exemplified by a now-infamous list of heroes.[108] Newton, Leonardo da Vinci, and Beethoven were included on Muller's list, but so were Marx and Lenin. Central planners could, of course, adopt a more long-term view and could make their choices only after soliciting the views of experts and the general public.

A third and mediating alternative for the selection of genetic enhancements is local initiative, often by parents, with a central veto to avoid excesses. Glover calls this proposal a mixed system. Why does Glover include a central veto in this system? He is concerned chiefly about the possibility of parents making idiosyncratic choices that might seriously harm the welfare of their children.

[S]ome parental choices would be disturbing. If parents chose characteristics likely to make their children unhappy, or likely to reduce their abilities, we might feel that the children should be protected against this. (Imagine parents belonging to some extreme religious sect, who wanted their children to have a religious symbol as a physical mark on their face, and who wanted them to be unable to read, as a protection against their faith being corrupted.) Those of us who support restrictions protecting children from parental harm after birth . . . are likely to support protecting children from being harmed by their parents' genetic choices.[109]

A second important policy question is how enhancement technologies, if and when they exist, will be allocated within the societies that have access to them. Answers to this question will roughly parallel the answers given in current biocthical debates about the allocation of health care resources.[110] Libertarian social philosophers like Robert Nozick accent the importance of individual freedom and adopt a free-market approach to the allocation of all social goods, presumably including genetic enhancement technologies. On this view, justice means:

From each according to what he chooses to do, to each according to what he makes for himself (perhaps with the contracted aid of others) and what others choose to do for him and choose to give him of what they've been given previously (under this maxim) and haven't yet expended or transferred.[111]

A possible objection to this proposal is that it might tend to reinforce and even accentuate existing socioeconomic differences. In other words, the only people allowed to shop in the genetic supermarket would be those who have enough money to buy groceries.

An alternative approach would be to allocate enhancement technologies to those who most need them, the least-well-off members of a society. With the physical and intellectual enhancements, the value of this compensatory approach to the least-well-off is clear. Genetic enhancements could help them to overcome the vagaries of the so-called *natural lottery* and, at least in some cases, to approach the level of species-typical functioning. In this approach, the long-term tendency of the system would be to reduce the physical and intellectual differences between the best-off and the worst-off. However, this approach to physical and intellectual enhancement would undoubtedly involve limitations on the liberty of the best-off, as well as the transfer of property, presumably through taxation, from the best-off to the worst-off. Moral enhancement of the "neediest" would be a tricky proposition, at best; it would require scrupulous attention to due process in order to avoid the stigmatization and attempted modification of unconventional but harmless attitudes and patterns of life. At the same time, however, we think that many people who are uncontrollably impulsive or violently aggressive would welcome the offer of moral enhancement by genetic means. (Recall, for example, the aggressive males in the Dutch kindred whose violent behavior was discussed earlier in this chapter.)[112] Those who are best-off in qualities like agreeableness or friendliness would presumably be quite willing to contribute to the provision of moral enhancement to the morally worst-off.

A third alternative would be to distribute genetic enhancements, or at least certain kinds of genetic enhancements, equally to all the members of a society. If this alternative were implemented, the long-term trend of the intervention would be to maintain current differences between the best-off and the worst-off but to improve the lot of everyone compared to his or her past lot. In addition, this policy would generally have the effect of improving the situation of the enhanced society vis-à-vis other societies that could not afford or did not choose to adopt the particular enhancement.

Toward a Moral Judgment about Genetic Enhancement

At the beginning of this discussion, we want to reiterate that genetic intervention is only one of several methods for improving the human condition. Social programs to help the least-well-off members of society, action to protect the environment from degradation, new technologies like personal computers, and cultural changes like increased appreciation for the diversity of human beings all have important roles to play. Even within the health care and public health spheres, it is possible that nongenetic approaches will in the short run, or even in the long run, be more cost-effective than gene-based approaches to reducing the disease burden of human beings. In this chapter we have attempted to explore several ways in which genetic enhancement could potentially benefit human beings. We continue to think that genetic technologies will provide one method for improving the human condition. Given the relatively early stage of development in the genetic technologies, it is too early to make any reliable predictions about how important these technologies can be or will be in the next several centuries.

In our judgment, health-related physical enhancements by genetic means are morally justifiable in principle. For example, the improvement of the human immune system so that it would be more adept at warding off disease and so that it would retain its youthful vigor as people age would seem to us to be a net benefit for the human race. This enhancement would help to ensure that its recipients are able to enjoy a normal life-span with a lower probability of contracting a life-threatening infection or cancer. If such an enhancement were widely disseminated, it would have the effect of gradually changing the normal range for health and disease. In other words, species-typical functioning would become a more dynamic notion and would gradually improve vis-à-vis at least some diseases.

We also think that intellectual genetic enhancements that allow people who fall below the normal range to achieve functioning within the normal range are ethically acceptable. For example, if a safe and reliable gene-based method for substantially improving the mental functioning of a moderately retarded young person were available, many benevolent parents would, we think, welcome this intervention as a means to help their child enjoy a more nearly normal life. Conceptually, this kind of improvement would simultaneously be enhancement and remediation, as we have noted. This type of action by parents seems to us to be qualitatively different from an attempt to give a child who is already in or above the normal range a competitive edge through intellectual genetic enhancement.[113]

More controversial, but still morally justifiable in our view, would be the use of moral enhancement for violent sociopaths—provided that such sociopaths freely consented to the intervention. The criteria for sociopathic behavior would need to be carefully drawn so that prophets, dissidents, whistleblowers, and other nonconformists would not be branded as sociopaths. We have in mind people who, because of their genes or their social development or a combination of the two factors, repeatedly act with great cruelty—raping, torturing, and murdering—and who seem to feel no remorse for their actions. The attempt to bring the thinking, feeling, and acting of such sociopaths within the normal range of human behavior would again be an attempt at remediation, which in this case might also be called rehabilitation. Some sociopaths would probably reject the offer of gene-mediated moral enhancement, but others might, at the deepest level, regret that they are as they are and might accept the offer of such enhancement.

The remaining types of genetic enhancements—non-health-related physical enhancements and intellectual and moral enhancements for persons who already are functioning within the normal range—seem to us to be more problematic. There are two principal difficulties that are likely to attach to these new technological possibilities in these contexts. The first difficulty is what might be called a new form of child abuse. As we have noted, even benevolent parents might go too far in the effort to enhance the physical or intellectual capabilities of their children, approving genetic modifications that are clearly not in the best interests of their children. However, even in this high-technology sphere there may be social policies that could be adopted to protect children from serious abuse—that is, to set limits on the range of parental discretion.[114] Such limits are in place, either in law or by custom, in other spheres like education, sexual intimacy, movie attendance, the use of illegal drugs, and the consumption of alcohol.

A more fundamental problem to be faced regarding genetic enhancements that are not health-related and nonremedial is the allocation of these enhancements. Earlier in this chapter we reviewed several possible schemes for distribution. This is one of the few questions discussed in this book on which we authors disagree. To one of us (J.G.P.), individual liberty is such an important feature of both morality and social and political life that it should only be interfered with to protect the defenseless—for example, children—from serious harm.[115] To the other author (L.W.), the long-term goal of reducing the gap between the best- and worst-off members of society is preeminently important, both as a sign of respect for the dignity of all human beings and as a means for reducing social conflict. Thus, our diverging social and political philosophies would lead us to two different proposals for allocating genetic enhancements.

What conception of health underlies the analysis of this chapter and the judgments about genetic enhancement that we have reached? For the most part, we have relied on the closely related notions of the normal range and species-typical functioning. Especially in our discussions of remediation, we have used the metaphor of moving from below the mean toward the mean. However, we have also advocated changing the normal range or species-typical functioning for the better, for example, through improvements in the human immune system. We would, in fact, be pleased to see improvements in human health such that everyone could enjoy a life free of disease and resultant disability until the end of his or her normal life-span. At the same time, however, we have carefully avoided the language and the goal of perfectionism or utopianism. In the sphere of physical genetic enhancement, we are not sure that immortality is a desirable goal. In the realm of intellectual and moral enhancement, we have advocated remediation in some circumstances, and we are open to gradual improvements, appropriately distributed, in other human characteristics. We do not think, however, that there is one ideal or perfect way to be or to act, in the intellectual and moral spheres. There are certain intellectual and moral characteristics or traits that are clearly undesirable and dysfunctional, and we have no hesitation in advocating that people be assisted in overcoming these characteristics and traits. While there may a certain general vision of the good society and the well-functioning human being that guides our analysis and helps us to identify which changes are in fact improvements, we do not have in mind, nor do we aspire to have the human race evolve toward, a perfect society or ideal human beings.

In conclusion, we should note that a particular perspective on human nature clearly underlies our moral judgments about genetic enhancement. We are dissatisfied with and critical of certain aspects of the human condition as we see it reflected in the world around us and as we experience it. In the physical sphere, we regard disease and disability as evils that should be overcome as quickly and efficiently as possible. In the intellectual and moral sphere we have also identified serious problems that should be addressed in multiple ways, one of which is through the judicious use of genetic technologies. We think that a certain dissatisfaction with human nature as it has developed and as we have inherited it is a prerequisite for intervention to improve human nature. Also implicit in the notion of genetic enhancement is a dynamic rather than a static view of human nature. While there are historical and evolutionary reasons for human nature's being as it is, we do not view the human race as being fated to accept the current state of affairs. Rather, we accept the possibility of change in human nature and have tried to argue for the ethical acceptability of certain kinds of planned changes in the characteristics of future human beings. In our view, such genetic enhancements are an important part of the overall task of attempting to provide a better life and a better world to our descendants.

Public Attitudes toward Genetic Enhancement

What does the United States public think about the possibility of enhancing human capabilities by genetic means? Two snapshots of U.S. public opinion have been taken, one in 1986 and the other in 1992. The Louis Harris organization conducted both surveys, by telephone, using identical questions with a cross-sectional sample of 1,273 (1986) and 1,000 (1992) respondents. Here is how the question was formulated: "How do you feel about scientists changing the makeup of human cells to . . . (e) improve the physical characteristics that children would inherit or (f) improve the intelligence level that children would inherit—would you strongly approve, somewhat approve, somewhat disapprove, or strongly disapprove?"[116]

For the physical enhancements, a slight majority of respondents disapproved. The precise figures from 1986 and 1992 (1986 in parentheses) are shown in Table 4-1.[117]

Table 4-1. Attitudes Toward Genetic Manipulation to Improve Physical Characteristics of Children

Strongly Approve	Somewhat Approve	Somewhat Disapprove	Strongly Disapprove	Not Sure
16% (16%)	27% (28%)	21% (23%)	33% (31%)	3 (3%)

1986 vs. (1992).

Table 4-2. Attitudes Toward Genetic Manipulation to Improve Intelligence of Children

Strongly Approve	Somewhat Approve	Somewhat Disapprove	Strongly Disapprove	Not Sure
17% (18%)	25% (26%)	20% (22%)	35% (31%)	3 (2%)

1992 vs. (1986).

The largest group of respondents, by far, strongly disapproved of this proposal. However, 43–44% of the respondents either strongly approved or somewhat approved of physical enhancements.

For intellectual enhancement the pattern of responses was quite similar (Table 4-2).[118] Again the largest group of respondents strongly disapproved. However, 42–44% of respondents either strongly approved or somewhat approved.

From these survey results we conclude that a slight majority of U.S. citizens are opposed to genetic enhancement in principle. At the same time a substantial minority are open to the idea of genetic enhancement. The percentages of respondents approving or disapproving will perhaps change over time, although the figures remained remarkably stable during the 5½ years between these two surveys. The percentages approving and disapproving could also vary with specific types of physical or intellectual enhancements.

Expert Opinion on Genetic Enhancement

Since most of the 28 policy statements on gene therapy identified in Chapter 2 presuppose a medical framework, they do not explicitly discuss genetic enhancement. Interestingly, none of the statements consider health-related genetic enhancements. The few statements that mention genetic enhancement as a general topic judge it to be ethically unacceptable. Typical rejections of genetic enhancement by advisory committees in the United Kingdom and Canada follow:

> We are firmly of the opinion that gene therapy should be directed to alleviating disease in individual patients, although wider applications may soon call for attention. In the present state of knowledge any attempt by gene modification to change human traits not associated with disease would not be acceptable.[119]

•   •   •

The Commission recommends that. . . . **No research involving the alteration of DNA for enhancement purposes be permitted or funded in Canada**.[120]

Conclusion

Genetic enhancement is without question the most controversial potential application of new genetic knowledge and techniques. Formidable technical obstacles face any effort to employ genetic technology in this way. However, at some point in the near or more distant future, the technical capability to enhance at least some human characteristics will be developed. Our goal in this chapter has been to distinguish among three principal categories of possible enhancement—physical, intellectual, and moral. Within the category of physical enhancements we have drawn a further distinction between enhancements that are health-related and those that are not. Toward the end of the chapter we have ventured to reach ethical judgments on several possible applications of genetic enhancement. If we have stimulated readers to think about these possibilities in a calm and rational way and to reach their own moral judgments about them, we will have accomplished our mission in writing the chapter.

Notes

1. Richard D. Palmiter et al., "Dramatic Growth of Mice That Develop from Eggs Microinjected with Metallothionein-Growth Hormone Fusion Gene," *Nature* 300(5893): 611–615; 16 December 1982; Richard D. Palmiter et al., "Metallothionein-Human GH Fusion Genes Stimulate Growth of Mice," *Science* 222(4625): 809–814; 18 November 1983; Robert E. Hammer et al., "Expression of Human Growth Hormone-Releasing Factor in Transgenic Mice Results in Increased Somatic Growth," *Nature* 315(6018): 413–416; 30 May 1985.

2. Palmiter et al., "Dramatic Growth".

3. Palmiter et al., "Metallothionein-Human GH Fusion Genes"; Hammer et al., op. cit.

4. Palmiter et al. (note 3), p. 814.

5. Hammer et al., op. cit.

6. President's Commission for the Study of Ethical Problems in Medicine and Biomedical and Behavioral Research, *Splicing Life: A Report on the Social and Ethical Issues of Genetic Engineering with Human Beings* (Washington, DC: The Commission, November 1982), p. 45; Zsolt Harsanyi, vice president of DNA sciences, E. F. Hutton and Co., testifying before the U.S. Congress, House, Committee on Science and Technology, Subcommitte on Investigations and Oversight, *Human Genetic Engineering*, Hearings, 97th Congress, 2d Session, 16–18 November 1982, p. 225; Bernard D. Davis, "Cells and Souls," *New York Times*, June 28, 1983, p. A27. See also the testimony of David Jackson, vice president and chief scientific officer at Genex Corporation, testifying before the U.S. Congress, *Human Genetic Engineering*, op. cit., p. 193.

7. President's Commission, *Splicing Life*, p. 45; Harsanyi, in U.S. Congress, *Human Genetic Engineering*, op. cit., p. 225; Davis, op. cit.; Jackson, in U.S. Congress, *Human Genetic Engineering*, p. 193; Eve K. Nichols, *Human Gene Therapy* (Cambridge, MA: Harvard University Press, 1988), p. 12. See also Jonathan Glover, *What Sort of People Should There Be?* (New York: Penguin Books, 1988) and Ted Howard and Jeremy Rifkin, *Who Should Play God?* (New York: Dell, 1977), p. 132.

8. Theodore Kurtz, "An ACE for Hypertension," *Nature* 353(6344): 499; 10 October 1991.

9. Nichols, op. cit.

10. John Lantos et al., "Ethical Issues In Growth Hormone Therapy," *JAMA* 261(7): 1020–1024; 17 February 1989. No randomized, controlled study of the effects of GH

administration on non–GH-deficient children has ever been performed (personal communication from John Lantos, May 1995).

11. Sandy Rovner, "The Great American Sleep Debt," Health section, *Washington Post*, January 12, 1993, p. 9. See also United States, National Commission on Sleep Disorders Research, *Wake Up, America: A National Sleep Alert: Report*, Volume 1: *Executive Summary and Executive Report* (Washington, DC: The Commission, January 1993).

12. Bob Condor, "The Body Clock," *Chicago Tribune*, October 31, 1994, Section 5, page 1; personal communication from Charmane Eastman, January 12, 1995.

13. Michael Stroh, "Genes May Help Reset Circadian Clock," *Science News* 141(13): 196; 28 March 1992. See also Martin R. Ralph and Michael Menaker, "A Mutation of the Circadian System in Golden Hamsters," *Science* 241(4870): 1225–1227; 2 September 1988; and Martin R. Ralph et al., "Transplanted Suprachiasmatic Nucleus Determines Circadian Period," *Science* 247(4945): 975–978; 23 February 1990.

14. Joseph S. Takahashi, Lawrence H. Pinto, and Martha Hotz Vitaterna, "Forward and Reverse Genetic Approaches to Behavior in the Mouse," *Science* 264(5166): 1724–1733; 17 June 1994.

15. Ronald J. Konopka, "Genetics of Biological Rhythms in Drosophila," *Annual Review of Genetics* 21(1987): 227–236; and Jeffrey C. Hall and Charalambos P. Kyriacou, "Genetics of Biological Rhythms in Drosophila," *Advances in Insect Physiology* 22(1990): 221–298.

16. Miodrag Radulovacki, "Phenoxybenzamine and Bromocriptine Attenuate Need for REM Sleep in Rats," *Pharmacology, Biochemistry and Behavior* 14(3): 371–375; March 1981.

17. It has been pointed out to us that resetting the circadian clock does not replenish other physiological capabilities (Martin Eglitis, review of manuscript, April 27, 1995).

18. Thomas E. Johnson, "Increased Life-Span of *age-1* Mutants in *Caenorhabditis elegans* and Lower Gompertz Rate of Aging," *Science* 249(4971): 908–912; 24 August 1990.

19. Thomas E. Johnson and Gordon J. Lithgow, "The Search for the Genetic Basis of Aging: The Identification of Gerontogenes in the Nematode *Caenorhabditis elegans*," *Journal of the American Geriatrics Society* 40(9): 938; September 1992.

20. Jerry E. Bishop, *Wall Street Journal*, "Good News for Worms: Study Finds Genetic Clue to Aging in Nematode," August 24, 1990, p. B2.

21. Ronald Kotulak and Peter Gorner, "Fruit Flies Provide Hint on Aging," *Chicago Tribune*, February 9, 1992, Section 1, pp. 21, 26. See also the earlier paper by Michael R. Rose, "Laboratory Evolution of Postponed Senescence in *Drosophila melanogaster*," *Evolution* 38(5): 1004–1010; September 1984.

22. Kotulak and Gorner (note 21), p. 21 (quoting Michael Rose).

23. Ibid., p. 26 (citing an interview with Johnson).

24. Makoto Goto et al., "Genetic Linkage of Werner's Syndrome to Five Markers on Chromosome 8," *Nature* 355(6362): 735–738; 20 February 1992.

25. T.V.P. Bliss, "Maintenance Is Presynaptic," *Nature* 346(6286): 698–699; 23 August 1990; Michael Waldholz, "Japanese Scientists Isolate Brain Gene Used in Memory," *Wall Street Journal*, November 7, 1991, p. B5.

26. Koki Moriyoshi et al., "Molecular Cloning and Characterization of the Rat NMDA Receptor," *Nature* 354(6348): 31–37; 7 November 1991; Waldholz, op. cit. See also Mark L. Mayer, "NMDA Receptors Cloned at Last," *Nature* 354(6348): 16–17; November 1991.

27. Keshava N. Kumar, "Cloning of cDNA for the Glutamate-Binding Subunit of an NMDA Receptor Complex," *Nature* 354(6348): 70–73; 7 November 1991.

28. For a recent study of the molecular basis of learning and memory in another species, the fruit fly, see Ralph J. Greenspan, "Understanding the Genetic Construction of Behavior," *Scientific American* 272(4): 76–77; April 1995. For a report on research on spatial learning and remembering in mice conducted by Jeanne Wehner of the Institute for Behavioral Research in Boulder, Colorado, see Marcia Barinaga, "From Fruit Flies, Rats, Mice: Evidence of Genetic Influence," *Science* 264(5166): 1692–1693; 17 June 1994.

29. Barbara L. Schwartz et al., "Glycine Prodrug Facilitates Memory Retrieval in Humans," *Neurology* 41(9): 1341–1343; September 1991. The study authors point out that milacemide may have improved memory retrieval by increasing arousal or attention rather than by specifically interacting with NMDA receptors but suggest that their study provides further evidence, when combined with evidence from other studies, that NMDA receptors are important in learning and memory.

30. Jill Murrell et al., "A Mutation in the Amyloid Precursor Protein Associated with Hereditary Alzheimer's Disease," *Science* 254(5028): 97–99; 4 October 1991; E.H. Corder et al., "Gene Dose of Apolipoprotein E Type 4 Allele and the Risk of Alzheimer's Disease in Late Onset Families," *Science* 261(5123): 921–923; 13 August 1993.

31. Murrell et al., ibid., p. 98.

32. Robert Plomin, Michael J. Owen, and Peter McGuffin, "The Genetic Basis of Complex Behaviors," *Science* 264(5166): 1736; 17 June 1994.

33. Corder et al., op. cit., pp. 922–923; Plomin et al., op. cit., p. 1737.

34. U.S., President's Commission, *Splicing Life* (note 6), p. 45; Jackson in U.S. Congress, *Human Genetic Engineering* (note 6), p. 193.

35. Martin Hooper et al., "HPRT-deficient (Lesch-Nyhan) Mouse Embryos Derived from Germline Colonization by Cultured Cells," *Nature* 326(6110): 292–295; 19 March 1987.

36. Jeremy Cherfas, "Molecular Biology Lies Down with the Lamb," *Science*, 249 (4965): 124–126; 13 July 1990. According to Cherfas, Hooper and his colleagues used homologous recombination in embryonic stem cells to transfer hypoxanthine-guanine-phosphoribosyltransferase (HPRT) genes into the germ lines of mice, a procedure that has been called gene surgery or gene targeting.

37. Burr Eichelman, "Bridges from the Animal Laboratory to the Study of Violent or Criminal Individuals," in Sheilagh Hodgins, ed., *Mental Disorder and Crime* (Newbury Park, CA: Sage Publications, 1993), pp. 194–195.

38. Frédéric Saudou et al., "Enhanced Aggressive Behavior in Mice Lacking 5–HT$_{1B}$ Receptor," *Science* 265(5180): 1875–1878; 23 September 1994. See also Marcia Barinaga, "The Mouse That Roared," *Science* 262(5137): 1211; 19 November 1993.

39. H.G. Brunner et al., "Abnormal Behavior Associated with a Point Mutation in the Structural Gene for Monoamine Oxidase A," *Science* 262(5133): 578–580; 22 October 1993; see also H.G. Brunner et al., "X-Linked Borderline Mental Retardation with Prominent Behavioral Disturbance: Phenotype, Genetic Localization, and Evidence for Disturbed Monoamine Metabolism," *American Journal of Human Genetics* 52(6): 1032–1039; June 1993.

40. On the general problem of reductionism in human genetics, see Evelyn Shuster, "Determinism and Reductionsim: A Greater Threat Because of the Human Genome Project?" in George J. Annas and Sherman Elias, eds., *Gene Mapping: Using Law and Ethics as Guides* (New York: Oxford University Press, 1992), pp. 115–127; and A. Lippman, "Led (Astray) by Genetic Maps: The Cartography of the Human Genome and Health Care," *Social Science and Medicine* 35(12): 1469–1476; December 1992.

41. On Lysenkoism in the Soviet Union, see Daniel J. Kevles, *In the Name of Eugenics: Genetics and the Social Uses of Human Heredity* (Berkeley, CA: University of California Press, 1985), pp. 187–188; and Elof Axel Carlson, *Genes, Radiation, and Society: The Life and Work of H. J. Muller* (Ithaca, NY: Cornell University Press, 1981), pp. 219–234.

42. See Robert N. Proctor, *Racial Hygiene: Medicine Under the Nazis* (Cambridge, MA: Harvard University Press, 1988).

43. Science Service was a private organization based in Washington, DC, that sought to distibute accurate, up-to-date information about science to newspapers and radio networks. The organization was founded in 1921; its trustees were nominated by three scientific groups—the National Academy of Sciences, the National Research Council, and the American Association for the Advancement of Science—and two newpaper groups. Soon after its founding, the organization began to produce a news service for newspapers. Beginning in 1922, Science Service also published a weekly magazine, *Science News Letter*. In 1966 the name of the weekly was changed to *Science News*. See Watson Davis, "The Rise of Scientific Understanding," *Science* 108(2801): 239–246; 3 September 1948.

44. "Social Biology and Population Improvement," *Nature* 144(3646): 521–522; 16 September, 1939.

45. Ibid., p. 521. The tripartite distinction among physical, intellectual, and moral enhancements was already implicit in Muller's 1935 book, *Out of the Night: A Biologist's View of the Future* (New York: Vanguard Press). See esp. pp. 84–86.

46. *Perspectives in Biology and Medicine* 3(1): 1–43; Autumn 1959.

47. Ibid., pp. 37–38.

48. Ibid., p. 38.

49. Ibid., p. 22.

50. In his imaginative philosophical book *What Sort of People Should There Be?* (note 7), Jonathan Glover also discusses several specific genetic enhancements. His primary focus is on intellectual and moral enhancements. See especially pp. 179–186.

51. Both the B cells (which produce antibodies against viruses and other pathogens) and the T cells (which identify and attack pathogens) seem to be primed by immunizations. See Ivan M. Roitt, *Immunology* (3rd ed.; St. Louis: Mosby, 1993), Chapter 15.

52. For a lively discussion of nongenetic technologies for performance enhancement see Michael H. Shapiro, "The Technology of Perfection: Performance Enhancement and the Control of Attributes," *Southern California Law Review* 65(1): 11–113; November 1991.

53. In our view, morally relevant distinctions can be drawn between cosmetic surgery and orthodontic treatment in children, although we admit that the line is not always sharp and clear in particular cases.

54. See, for example, Norman Fost, "Banning Drugs in Sports: A Skeptical View," *Hastings Center Report* 16(4): 5–10; August 1986; and Thomas H. Murray, "Sports," in Warren T. Reich, ed.-in-chief, *Encyclopedia of Bioethics* (revised ed.; New York: Simon and Schuster Macmillan, 1995), Vol. V, pp. 2407–2410.

55. We acknowledge that similar concerns arise in nonsports competitive contexts— for example, cosmetic surgery for actors and actresses and other public figures. In the future, a parallel set of issues may arise for gene-mediated enhancements. However, the sports context seems to us to raise the issue of competitive fairness in a more direct and immediate way than the general social context does. On this point, see Hans Lenk, "Toward a Social Philosophy of Achievement and Athletics," in William Morgan and Klaus Meier, eds., *Philosophic Inquiry in Sport* (Champaign, IL: Human Kinetics Publishers, 1988), p. 393.

56. Jane E. Brody, "Discovering the Limits to Using Growth Hormone," *New York Times*, July 19, 1995, p. C8.

57. Ibid.

58. Ibid.

59. For a recent survey of sleep research, see J. Allan Hobson and Robert Stickgold, "The Conscious State Paradigm: A Neurocognitive Approach to Waking, Sleeping, and Dreaming," in Michael S. Gazzaniga, ed.-in-chief, *The Cognitive Neurosciences* (Cambridge, MA: MIT Press, 1995), pp. 1373–1389. See also John S. Antrobus and Mario Bertini, eds., *The Neuropsychology of Sleep and Dreaming* (Hillsdale, NJ: Lawrence Erlbaum Associates, 1992). According to Isaac Lewin and Jerome L. Singer, some neuropsychologists assign important roles to rapid-eye-movement (REM) sleep, which is associated with vivid dreams. Other neuropyschologists consider both REM and non-REM sleep to be nonessential carryovers from an earlier stage of evolution. On the latter view, the gradual abolition of the sleep-drive mechanism during further evolution would have no deleterious effects ("Psychological Effects of REM ('Dream') Deprivation upon Waking Mentation," in Steven J. Ellman and John S. Antrobus, eds., *The Mind in Sleep: Psychology and Psychophysiology* [2nd ed.; New York: John Wiley & Sons, 1991], esp. pp. 398–399 and 403–407).

60. On this point, see Leonard Hayflick, "Biological Aging Theories," in George L. Maddon, ed.-in-chief, *The Encyclopedia of Aging* (New York: Springer Publishing Company, 1987), pp. 64–68; and François Schächter, Daniel Cohen, and Tom Kirkwood, "Prospects for the Genetics of Human Longevity," *Human Genetics* 91(6): 519–526; July 1993.

61. See Leon Kass, "The Case for Mortality," *American Scholar* 52(2): 173–191; Spring 1983; and Daniel Callahan, *Setting Limits: Medical Goals in an Aging Society* (New York: Simon and Schuster, 1987); and Hans Jonas, "The Burden and Blessing of Mortality," *Hastings Center Report* 22(1): 34–40; January–February 1992.

62. See Albert Rosenfeld, *Prolongevity* (New York: Alfred A. Knopf, 1976); Bernice L. Neugarten and Robert J. Havighurst, eds., *Extending the Human Life Span: Social Policy and Social Ethics* (Washington, DC: U.S. Government Printing Office, 1977); Arthur Caplan, "The 'Unnaturalness' of Aging—A Sickness unto Death," in Arthur L. Caplan, et al., eds., *Concepts of Health and Disease* (Reading, MA: Addison-Wesley, 1981), pp. 725–737; and Timothy F. Murphy, "A Cure for Aging?" *Journal of Medicine and Philosophy* 11(3): 237–255; August 1986.

63. After writing this section, we discovered that two commentators on the ethics of genetic engineering, Peter Singer and Deane Wells, had advocated genetic intervention to allow human beings to live out the normal human life-span free of life-shortening disease but had not recommended genetic engineering to extend the normal life-span. See their "Genetic Engineering," in Erwin Edward, Sidney Gendin, and Lowell Kleiman, eds., *Ethical Issues in Scientific Research: An Anthology* (New York: Garland Publishing Company, 1994), pp. 307–320.

64. *The Future of Man* (New York: Mentor Books, 1961), p. 95.

65. *Social Philosophy and Policy* 8(1): 185; Autumn 1990. Footnote a reads as follows: "Some have written of menopause as a disease, indicating the need to use disease language in order to authorize desired medical interventions. Robert W. Kistner, The Menopause, *Clinical Obstetrics and Gynecology*, vol. 16 (December 1973), pp. 107–29."

66. Medawar, op. cit., p. 96.

67. Plomin et al. (note 32).

68. Ibid., p. 1736.

69. E.H. Corder et al. (note 30).

70. *The Descent of Man and Selection in Relation to Sex* (revised ed.; New York: D. Appleton and Company, 1896), Part I, Chapter II (pp. 27–28). Footnote a reads: "'Variation of Animals and Plants under Domestication,' vol. ii, chap. xii." Footnote b reads: "'Hereditary Genius: an Inquiry into Its Laws and Consequences,' 1869."

71. London: Murray, 1859, p. 213.

72. Glayde Whitney, "A Contextual History of Behavioral Genetics," in Martin E. Hahn et al., eds., *Developmental Behavior Genetics: Neural, Biometrical, and Evolutionary Approaches* (New York: Oxford University Press, 1990), pp. 15–18.

73. New York: John Wiley & Sons, 1960.

74. Ibid., p. ix.

75. John Horgan, "Genes and Crime," *Scientific American* 268(2): 122–131; February 1993.

76. Paul R. Billings, Jonathan Beckwith, and Joseph S. Alper, "The Genetic Analysis of Human Behavior: A New Era?" *Social Science and Medicine* 35(3): 227–238; August 1992.

77. "The Emanuel Miller Memorial Lecture 1993: Genetic Research and Identification of Environmental Influences," *Journal of Child Psychology and Psychiatry* 35(5): 822; July 1994.

78. For recent surveys of the field see Plomin et al. (note 32); and Richard J. Rose, "Genes and Human Behavior," *Annual Review of Psychology* 46(1995): 625–654.

79. For a recent attempt to explore the roles of nature and of nurture in psychology, see Robert Plomin and Gerald E. McClearn, eds., *Nature, Nurture, and Psychology* (Washington, DC: American Psychological Association, 1993). For help in locating the literature on behavioral genetics, we are deeply indebted to Ms. Teresa Doksum, who prepared an "Annotated Bibliography of Behavioral Genetics" (February 1995) for the National Institutes of Health–Department of Energy Working Group on Ethical, Legal, and Social Implications (ELSI) of the Human Genome Project.

80. United States, Office of Technology Assessment (OTA), *New Developments in Biotechnology—Background Paper: Public Perceptions of Biotechnology* (Washington, DC: U.S. Government Printing Office, May 1987); and March of Dimes (MOD) Birth Defects Foundation, *Genetic Testing and Gene Therapy Survey: Questionnaire and Responses* (White Plains, NY: March of Dimes Birth Defects Foundation, September 1992).

81. See, for example, the following introductions to the neurosciences: Alan Frazer, Perry B. Molinoff, and Andrew Winokur, eds., *Biological Bases of Brain Function and Disease* (New York: Raven Press, 1994); John E. Dowling, *Neurons and Networks: An Introduction to Neuroscience* (Belknap Press of Harvard University Press, 1992); and Eric R. Kandel, James H. Schwartz, and Thomas M. Jessell, eds., *Principles of Neural Science* (New York: Elsevier, 1991).

82. On long-term memory, in general, see Joaquin M. Fuster, *Memory in the Cerebral Cortex: An Empirical Approach to Neural Networks in the Human and Nonhuman Primate* (Cambridge, MA: MIT Press, 1995), pp. 12–22, 211–216; and Yadin Dudai, *The Neurobiology of Memory: Concepts, Findings, Trends* (New York: Oxford University Press, 1989), pp. 119–138, 247–265. See also Larry R. Squire, ed.-in-chief, *Encyclopedia of Learning and Memory* (New York: Macmillan, 1992).

83. James L. McGaugh, "Enhancing Cognitive Performance," *Southern California Law Review* 65(1): 383–395; November 1991; Richard J. Rose, op. cit. (note 78), pp. 643–644.

84. On this scale, see the following works: Alan S. Kaufman, *Intelligent Testing with the WISC-III* (New York: Wiley, 1994); and George Frank, *The Wechsler Enterprise: An*

Assessment of the Development, Structure and Use of the Wechsler Tests of Intelligence (New York: Pergamon Press, 1983).

85. See, for example, Robert Plomin and Richard Rende, "Human Behavioral Genetics," in Mark R. Rosenzweig and Lyman W. Porter, eds., *Annual Review of Psychology* 42 (1991), pp. 162–163; Stephanie D. Castro; J.C. DeFries; and David W, Fulker, "Multivariate Genetic Analysis of Wechsler Intelligence Scale for Children—Revised (WISC—R) Factors," *Behavior Genetics* 25(1): 25–32; January 1995; Plomin et al., op. cit., p. 1734; Richard J. Rose, op. cit., pp. 627–630; Lon R. Cardon, "Genetics of Specific Cognitive Abilities," in Plomin and McClearn, *Nature, Nurture, and Psychology* (note 79), pp. 99–120. One of the two authors of this book (J.G.P.) is skeptical about the usefulness of standardized tests of cognitive function and about the correlations that are asserted by behavioral scientists between genetic factors and what is measured by standardized tests.

86. Castro, et al. (note 85).

87. Rose, op. cit., pp. 631–632; Plomin et al., p. 1736.

88. Glover (note 7), pp. 179–181.

89. A distinct issue, also a matter that merits discussion, is whether society is too preoccupied with cognitive ability and not sufficiently concerned, for example, with moral qualities.

90. In other words, just as parents are at liberty to employ *environmental* measures to enhance the overall academic achievement of their children, so parents should be free, within limits, within reasonable limits, to select *genetic* means to achieve the same goal.

91. A Symposium on the Genetics of Criminal and Antisocial Behaviour was held in London on February 14–16, 1995. The symposium was sponsored by the Ciba Foundation. The papers presented at the symposium were published in early 1996. See Gregory R. Bock and Jamie A. Goode, eds., *Genetics of Criminal and Antisocial Behaviour* (Chichester and New York: Wiley, 1996).

92. H.G. Brunner et al., "X-Linked Borderline Mental Retardation" (note 39), p. 1035; see also H.G. Brunner et al., "Abnormal Behavior" (note 39), pp. 578–580.

93. Brunner et al., "Abnormal Behavior," p. 579.

94. Eichelman (note 37), pp. 198–200.

95. Ibid., pp. 194–195.

96. See the recent survey of this evidence in Albert J. Reiss, Jr., and Jeffrey A. Roth, eds., *Understanding and Preventing Violence* (Washington, DC: National Academy Press, 1993), pp. 115–121. For a study that produced aggression in mice by *knocking out* one type of receptor for serotonin, see Saudou et al. (note 38).

97. Thomas J. Bouchard, "Genes, Environment, and Personality," *Science* 264(5166): 1700–1701; 17 June 1994. The five super factors are *extraversion, neuroticism, conscientiousness, agreeableness,* and *openness.*

98. Ibid., p. 1700.

99. Plomin et al., op. cit., p. 1738.

100. Engelhardt (note 65), p. 188.

101. Ibid. Footnote a: "For an account of the sociobiological basis of male aggressiveness, see F.B. Livingstone, The Effects of Warfare on the Biology of the Human Species, ed. M. Fried, M. Harris, and R. Murphy, *War: The Anthropology of Armed Conflict and Aggression* (Garden City: Natural History Press, 1967), pp. 3–15. See also Donald Symons, *The Evolution of Human Sexuality* (New York: Oxford University Press, 1979), pp. 144–58. For an ethnographic study of violence, see Napoleon A. Chagnon, *Yanomano: The Fierce People* (2nd ed.; New York: Hold, Rinehart and Winston, 1977)." Footnote b: "These prudential considerations regarding mass destruction would play a role in addition to other

moral judgements that one would want to make regarding homicidal proclivities even under natural circumstances." Footnote c: "For a description of some of the syndromes I have in mind, see Vernon H. Mark and Frank R. Ervin, *Violence and the Brain* (New York: Harper & Row, 1970). The authors indicate their view that some dispositions to extreme violence may have important genetic components."

102. Glover, op. cit., pp. 181–182.

103. Ibid., p. 184.

104. Samuel Taylor Coleridge, *Biographia Literaria*, Chapter 14.

105. Glover, op. cit., p. 184.

106. See, for example, Karl Rahner, "The Experiment with Man: Theological Observations on Man's Self-Manipulation," in his *Theological Investigations*, Vol. IX, translated by Graham Harrison (New York: Herder and Herder, 1972), pp. 205–224. A German version of this essay was published in 1966.

107. Robert Nozick, *Anarchy, State and Utopia* (New York: Basic Books, 1974), p. 315.

108. Muller, *Out of the Night* (note 45), p. 113.

109. Glover, op. cit., p. 48.

110. For a recent survey of competing conceptions of justice and their possible implications for health care allocation, see Tom L. Beauchamp and James F. Childress, *Principles of Biomedical Ethics* (4th ed.; New York: Oxford University Press, 1994), esp. pp. 326–394.

111. Nozick, op. cit., p. 160.

112. See pp. 123–124.

113. This qualitative difference does not, however, mean that one action is applauded and the other condemned.

114. William Gardner points out that regulation of parental decisions regarding genetic enhancement will be quite difficult. See his interesting essay, "Can Human Genetic Enhancement Be Prohibited?," *Journal of Medicine and Philosophy* 20(1): 65–84; February 1995.

115. Julie Gage Palmer adopts this position in part because of her general skepticism about large social institutions, especially the state.

116. OTA, p. 105.

117. OTA, p. 73; MOD, p. 3.

118. OTA, p. 73; MOD, p. 3.

119. United Kingdom, Committee on the Ethics of Gene Therapy, *Report* (London: Her Majesty's Stationery Office, January 1992), p. 22.

120. Royal Commission on New Reproductive Technologies, *Proceed with Care* (2 vols.; Ottawa: Minister of Government Services Canada, 1993), Vol. 2, p. 945. Emphasis in original text.

5

Public Policy
on Human
Gene Therapy

During the early and middle 1960s a few scientists, theologians, and philosophers discussed the genetic engineering of human beings.[1] However, in the United States it was only in 1967 that the modern debate about human gene therapy as an application of molecular biology began. In August of that year Marshall Nirenberg of the National Heart Institute published an editorial in *Science* entitled, "Will Society Be Prepared?" After reviewing recent advances in biochemical genetics, Nirenberg wrote:

The point which deserves special emphasis is that man may be able to program his own cells with synthetic information long before he will be able to assess adequately the long-term consequences of such alterations, long before he will be able to formulate goals, and long before he can resolve the ethical and moral problems which will be raised. When man becomes capable of instructing his own cells, he must refrain from doing so until he has sufficient wisdom to use this knowledge for the benefit of mankind. I state this problem well in advance of the need to resolve it, because decisions concerning the application of this knowledge must ultimately be made by society, and only an informed society can make such decisions wisely.[2]

A few months later another eminent scientist, Joshua Lederberg of Stanford University, wrote a letter of response to the Nirenberg editorial. Lederberg's letter, entitled "Dangers of Reprogramming Cells," was published in the October 20th issue of *Science*. Excerpts follow.

In an editorial, "Will society be prepared?" (11 Aug., p. 633), Nirenberg wrote about the prospects of molecular genetics . . .

No subject of policy is more important than this, and it deserves the most critical debate. There is some danger that, whether so intended or not, Nirenberg's language could generate public misunderstandings that might undercut the very research needed to reach sufficient wisdom. His underlying concern, which I share, is that biological control might be used by a malevolent government to the peril of individual freedom.

· · ·

Our main concern must be to maximize the role of individual decision. This could be defeated by overenthusiastic policing of personal initiative and experimentation as well as by premature positive measures imposed by the state.[3]

Public policymakers in the United States first showed signs of interest in gene therapy the following year. On February 8th, 1968, Senator Walter Mondale of Minnesota introduced Joint Resolution 145, designed "to establish a Commission on Health Science and Society." In his accompanying statement Senator Mondale remarked:

Genetic intervention also raises moral and ethical questions of the most profound magnitude.

Geneticists, such as Dr. Lederberg, stress that they are not going to change the bodies of any existing people. But if there is a possibility for the future, we should be thankful that we have many years to think and plan. I am happy that I do not have to think about deciding which kinds of people would represent "perfecting the race" through genetic chemistry and which would not.[4]

When the hearings on Mondale's proposal were held in March and early April of 1968, Arthur Kornberg and Joshua Lederberg were two of the early witnesses. Both were at pains to minimize the social hazards associated with recent advances in molecular biology. Indeed, when one reads the hearing record as a whole, it is clear that other issues received much greater emphasis than human genetic engineering or gene therapy. These issues included the definition of death, cardiac transplantation, the allocation and overall cost of renal dialysis, the prolongation of life, and research involving human subjects.

From the time of the hearings on the Mondale bill in 1968 to November of 1982, no attention was paid by the United States Congress to the specific topic of human gene therapy. In the sphere of genetics and molecular biology, two related topics dominated the national public-policy agenda during this period. The first was genetic testing and screening, particularly newborn screening for phenylketonuria (PKU) and population screening of African Americans for sickle cell anemia or sickle cell trait. These issues were confronted by the United States Congress in the National Sickle Cell Anemia Control Act (Public Law No. 92–294), enacted in 1972.[5] In the same year the Committee for the Study of Inborn Errors of Metabolism was appointed by the National Research Council and began working on guidelines for genetic testing and screening. The committee's report was published in 1975.[6] Even more visible in the 1970s was a second public-policy discussion—the debate about the potential biohazards of recombinant DNA research. This debate led to numerous Congressional hearings, especially in 1976 and 1977, and to proposals to establish a group not unlike the Nuclear Regulatory Commission to oversee laboratory research with recombinant DNA.[7] In the end, the National Institutes of Health forestalled federal legislation by establishing the Recombinant DNA Advisory Committee (RAC) in October 1974 and publishing guidelines for recombinant DNA research in 1976. The RAC initially reviewed all recombinant DNA research performed in institutions receiving federal funds for such research. In the late 1970s and early 1980s, as evidence accumulated to indicate that recombinant DNA research was safe, the review process for most types of such research devolved to local institutional biosafety committees.

The year 1980 marks the first clear appearance of the gene therapy issue in the U.S. public-policy arena. A few days after the U.S. Supreme Court decision that allowed the patenting of genetically engineered microorganisms (*Diamond v. Chakrabarty*[8]), the general secretaries of three major religious groups in the United States sent a letter to then-President Jimmy Carter. The letter read in part as follows:

June 20, 1980

We are rapidly moving into a new era of fundamental danger triggered by the rapid growth of genetic engineering. Albeit, there may be opportunity for doing good; the very term suggests the danger. Who shall determine how human good is best served when new life forms are being engineered? Who shall control genetic experimentation and its results which could have untold implications for human survival? Who will benefit and who will bear any adverse consequences, directly or indirectly?

These are not ordinary questions. These are moral, ethical, and religious questions. They deal with the fundamental nature of human life and the dignity and worth of the individual human being.

• • •

We believe, after careful investigation, that no government agency or committee is currently exercising adequate oversight or control, nor addressing the fundamental ethical questions in a major way. Therefore, we intend to request that President Carter provide a way for representatives of a broad spectrum of our society to consider these matters and advise the government on its necessary role.[9]

At its July 1980 meeting the President's Commission on Bioethics, midway through its first year of activity, considered the letter from the three religious leaders. The commission's initial response was to survey government agencies concerning their current activities in the genetic engineering arena and to contract for a review of this field. At its September 1980 meeting the commission heard from representatives of the federal agencies most actively involved in human genetics. The commissioners also heard testimony by several invited witnesses on the scientific prospects for and the ethical implications of human genetic engineering. In response, the commission decided to add a study of genetic engineering to its already-formidable list of mandated studies.[10]

Less than a month after the commission's decision, the *Los Angeles Times* broke the story of two unauthorized gene therapy studies that had been performed by Dr. Martin Cline of UCLA.[11] The studies had been conducted in July of 1980 with two thalassemia patients, one in Israel and one in Italy.[12] The public disclosure of Cline's studies led to an internal investigation by UCLA and an external investigation by an ad hoc committee appointed by the director of NIH. As the parallel investigations continued, two essays on gene therapy were published in the *New England Journal of Medicine*—one by W. French Anderson and John C. Fletcher entitled "Gene Therapy in Humans: When Is It Ethical to Begin?,"[13] the other by Karen E. Mercola and Martin J. Cline entitled "The Potentials of Inserting New Genetic Information."[14]

In February of 1981, UCLA concluded its investigation by asking Dr. Cline to resign his administrative position as chief of the Division of Hematology-Oncology within the Department of Medicine. In May of the same year the ad hoc NIH committee reported to NIH Director Fredrickson, with a recommendation that all of Dr. Cline's current grants be reviewed in light of his violation of federal human-subjects regulations and guidelines for recombinant DNA research. In addition, a copy of the committee's report was to be appended to all future grant applications submitted to NIH by Dr. Cline for a period of 3 years. One NIH institute terminated a grant to Dr. Cline, a second temporarily interrupted support for a large program project, and a third continued his funding.[15]

At the beginning of 1982, the primary focus of public-policy discussion regarding human genetic engineering shifted to Europe, and more specifically to the Parliamentary Assembly of the Council of Europe. Already in January of 1980 Mr. B. Elmquist, a Danish member of the Legal Affairs Committee, had requested that the assembly pass a "recommendation on the protection of humanity against genetic engineering."[16] Mr. Elmquist's request led, in turn, to a 2-day parliamentary hearing in Copenhagen, Denmark, on May 25th and 26th, 1981—about the same time as the public release of the NIH ad hoc committee report on Martin Cline's unauthorized experiments. A report based on this hearing was published in January 1982 under the title *Genetic Engineering: Risks and Chances for Human Rights*.[17] In the same month the Legal Affairs Committee of the assembly presented a report on genetic engineering and a draft recommendation to the full assembly.[18] On January 26th the Parliamentary Assembly adopted Recommendation 934 (1982), which asserted the right of every human being to "inherit a genetic pattern that has not been artificially changed."[19] At the same time, however, the assembly seemed to allow for the possibility of germ-line genetic intervention to prevent or cure disease. Thus, the right to a genetic inheritance that has not been artificially interfered with was acknowledged "except in accordance with certain principles which are recognised as being fully compatible with respect for human rights (as, for example, in the field of therapeutic applications)."[20] Recommendation 934 was the first statement on human genetic intervention by a governmental or quasi-governmental body.

In November of the same year, 1982, Congressman Albert Gore, Jr., convened 3 days of hearings on human genetic engineering. The hearings were initiated by the first public presentation of the *Splicing Life* report[21]—the final product of a 2-year study process undertaken by the President's Commission on Bioethics. In general, the report argued that no qualitatively new ethical and social questions were raised by somatic cell gene therapy. A concluding chapter of the report considered alternative mechanisms for overseeing human gene therapy in the future.

The 3-day hearing convened by Mr. Gore, chairman of the Subcommittee on Investigations and Oversight of the House Science and Technology Committee, provided an opportunity for scientists, clinicians, ethicists, and lawyers to comment on the state of the art in and the ethical and legal implications of human genetic intervention. A dramatic moment occurred on the third day of the hearing when Martin Cline testified about his unauthorized gene therapy studies of 1980 and asked Chairman Gore whether he would rather have an experienced clinician or an interdisciplinary committee make decisions about the health care of Mr. Gore's hypothetical 13-year-old child. Mr. Gore replied that he would want to be sure that what the clinician was proposing for the child "bore reference to the best science available" and was not "a procedure so experimental as to have no known chance of benefiting my child whatsoever."[22]

A constant refrain in the November 1982 hearings was Mr. Gore's question, "Do you think that there should be some kind of new government body or commission to oversee the development of human gene therapy?" Most witnesses answered in the affirmative.[23] Encouraged by these responses, Mr. Gore introduced a bill a few months later, H.R. 2788, that sought to establish "the President's Commission on the Human Applications of Genetic Engineering." This bill was introduced on April 27th, 1983, less than a month after the President's Commission on Bioethics had completed its work and gone out of existence.

Meanwhile, the chairman of the NIH Recombinant DNA Advisory Committee had received a copy of the *Splicing Life* report from the President's Commission and was considering whether and how the RAC might respond to that report. Of particular interest was the final chapter of the report and its discussion of alternative mechanisms for the early studies of gene therapy in human beings. One oversight mechanism explicitly discussed by the commission was a revised or reconstituted RAC.[24]

By early 1983 the NIH RAC had been functioning for 8 years. It had overseen and indeed regulated most recombinant DNA research in the United States in the 1970s through its guidelines. As the perceived risks of laboratory research with recombinant DNA had diminished, the RAC gradually relaxed the guidelines and turned its primary attention to newer issues like the use of recombinant DNA techniques to produce biological products (for example, insulin) and the deliberate release of recombinant DNA into the environment. While the RAC was an advisory committee within the National Institutes of Health and the Department of Health and Human Services, it was comprised primarily of members who were not federal employees, and its meetings were always held in public. Scientists and clinicians constituted the majority of members, but scientists sympathetic to Science for the People, as well as lawyers and ethicists, were also members of the committee. Within the scientific community the RAC and the NIH director in the latter half of the 1970s, Donald Fredrickson, were credited with having forestalled an overreaction by Congress in regulating recombinant DNA research.

At the April 1983 RAC meeting Chairman Robert Mitchell, a California attorney and Reagan administration appointee, asked RAC members how they wished to respond to the *Splicing Life* report of the president's commission. On April 11th, RAC members decided to establish a Working Group on a Response to the *Splicing Life* Report. At a meeting on June 24th the Working Group agreed to recommend to the RAC that it declare its readiness, in principle, to review gene therapy proposals when this technique was ready for human application.

The parent committee accepted this recommendation at its September meeting. It further asked the Working Group to suggest guidelines and review procedures for gene therapy. In December 1983 the Working Group held its second and final meeting. From this meeting there emerged the suggestion that an interdisciplinary working group or subcommittee of the RAC be appointed that would be familiar with both the scientific and the ethical and social issues surrounding gene therapy. An eight-member working group was suggested, to be comprised of two clinicians, two laboratory scientists, two ethicists, and two lawyers. At its February 1984 meeting the RAC accepted this additional recommendation. On April 26th, the NIH director, James Wyngaarden, concurred.

During the summer of 1984 the members of the initial Working Group on Human Gene Therapy were chosen. The appointment process was quite informal and involved several parts of NIH and numerous external consultants. By the end of the summer a 15-person working group was in place. Though the actual working group was slightly larger than the group originally envisioned by the RAC, it included approximately equal numbers of members from clinical medicine, laboratory science, ethics, and law. One of us (L.W.) had the privilege of chairing the working group.[25]

As the Working Group on Human Gene Therapy prepared for its first meeting in the fall of 1984, it was not clear that any new guidelines would be necessary for research in human gene therapy. The federal regulations regarding research with human subjects were quite detailed and explicit, and researchers now had, as well, the careful ethical analysis of the president's commission in its *Splicing Life* report. However, a subgroup of the Working Group that met in September 1984 concluded that some kind of guidance document for researchers would be helpful. The subgroup proceeded to prepare a 13-page document entitled "Points to Consider in the Design of Human Gene Therapy Protocols." This document was discussed and substantially revised at and after the first meeting of the full Working Group on Human Gene Therapy on October 12th, 1984.

Later in October the Working Group reported to the parent RAC, which encouraged the group to proceed with developing the "Points to Consider." After its November meeting, the Working Group was ready to present its document to the public. On January 22, 1985, the "Points to Consider in the Design and Submission of Human Somatic-Cell Gene Therapy Protocols" was published in the *Federal Register*.[26] After reviewing public comments on this draft, the Working Group published a second version of the "Points to Consider" in the August 19, 1985, issue of the *Federal Register*.[27] At its September 1985 meeting the parent committee accepted this version with minor modifications.

The "Points to Consider" ask researchers to respond to more than 100 specific questions if those questions apply to their protocols.[28] However, these many questions can be summarized in seven central questions.

1. What is the disease to be treated, and why is it a good candidate for gene therapy?
2. What alternative treatments are available for this disease?
3. What is the potential harm associated with the genetic intervention?
4. What is the potential benefit associated with the intervention?
5. What steps will be taken to ensure that participants in the study are selected in a manner that is fair to everyone who wants to take part in the study?
6. What steps will be taken to ensure that the consent of study participants is both informed and voluntary?
7. What steps will be taken to protect the privacy of participants and the confidentiality of medical information about them?

The first four questions deal with outcomes or consequences of a disease, alternative treatments, and the proposed genetic intervention. These questions can be related to what moral philosophers call the *principle of beneficence*. The fifth question relates most directly to fairness or equity and to the general principle of justice. The final two questions in the series inquire about the self-determination of participants in gene therapy research and implicitly refer to the general principle of respect for the autonomy of persons.[29]

During the entire year of 1985 the Working Group on Human Gene Therapy worked on the "Points to Consider" with a sense of urgency. The members of the group were convinced that the initial submission of a gene therapy protocol was imminent. In fact, it was only in April of 1987 that a prototype gene therapy protocol was submitted by W. French Anderson and his colleagues at the National Institutes of Health. This prototype, called "Human Gene Therapy: Preclinical Data Document," illustrated how a protocol designed to treat severe combined immune deficiency (SCID) would respond to the questions raised in "Points to Consider." The Working Group (now called the Human Gene Therapy Subcommittee) took the "Preclinical Data Document" seriously and conducted a full-scale review of the document in December 1987 as if it were in fact an actual clinical protocol.

The first actual protocol involving gene transfer into human subjects was submitted to the RAC 4 months later, in April 1988, by Steven A. Rosenberg, W. French Anderson, and their collaborators at NIH. However, this protocol involved the marking of cells by means of new genes so that the cells could be followed in the bodies of patients, rather than gene therapy in the strict sense. Nonetheless, the subcommittee decided to review the gene-marking study at its July 1988 meeting. A vigorous, and at times heated, discussion occurred between the researchers and some members of the subcommittee. It was clear that at least one member of the subcommittee did not think that enough preclinical work had been done to justify moving into human patients. Indeed, the subcommittee as a whole asked for additional data on several key points in the protocol as a precondition for its approval. After a somewhat stormy maiden voyage that involved RAC approval in October, deferral by the NIH director, further review and approval by the Human Gene Therapy Subcommittee in December, a mail ballot by RAC members, approval by the NIH director, and a lawsuit by the Foundation on Economic Trends, the gene-marking study was initiated in May 1989. The results of this study were published in the *New England Journal of Medicine* in August 1990.[30]

On March 30, 1990, the first gene therapy protocol was presented to the Human Gene Therapy Subcommittee by R. Michael Blaese, W. French Anderson, and NIH colleagues. The actual clinical protocol for gene therapy bore a striking resemblance to the "Preclinical Data Document" of 1987. Like the earlier prototype, the actual protocol sought to treat children with SCID by providing the missing gene that produces a critical enzyme, *adenosine deaminase*. Unlike the earlier prototype, which had proposed adding the gene to each child's bone marrow cells, the actual protocol envisioned adding the missing gene to white blood cells that could be removed from the child's body by a process similar to blood donation. After the white blood cells had been treated in the laboratory and the gene had been added to as many of them as possible, the cells would be returned to the child's body through an intravenous infusion.

In the actual review of this protocol, conducted by the Human Gene Therapy Subcommittee in June and July of 1990, two questions emerged as central. The first was whether an alternative therapy, treatment with a synthetic enzyme derived from cattle, was sufficiently effective to obviate the need for human gene therapy for SCID. The cost of the enzyme therapy was formidable—$4,000 for each weekly injection—yet the cost issue alone would not have been an adequate reason to proceed with gene therapy. More important for subcommittee members were the arguments by the researchers that the synthetic enzyme could provoke an immune response in children over the long run because of its origin in cattle and that some children do not benefit, at least over time, from the enzyme therapy. This gene therapy study was approved by the Human Gene Therapy Subcommittee on July 30th, 1990. At the same subcommittee meeting a second gene therapy study was also approved. This study, reviewed by the subcommittee for the first time in July, sought to treat patients with malignant melanoma by means of white blood cells that carry the gene for tumor neciosis factor, which attacks and shrinks cancers. The cancer protocol was submitted by Steven Rosenberg and his associates. On July 31st, the parent committee also approved these first two gene therapy protocols. As noted in chapter 2, the first patient treated in the Blaese–Anderson protocol received her initial infusion of genetically modified cells in September of 1990.

During the years 1990–1995 a total of 100 gene therapy protocols have been submitted to and approved by the NIH Recombinant DNA Advisory Committee. The target diseases in these protocols have been the following:

Cancers of various types: 63
HIV infection/AIDS: 12
Genetic diseases: 22
Other diseases: 3
       Rheumatoid arthritis: 1
       Peripheral artery disease: 1
       Arterial restenosis: 1

The genetic diseases that have been approached by means of gene therapy have included cystic fibrosis (12 protocols), Gaucher disease (type I) (3 protocols), SCID (1), familial hypercholesterolemia (1), alpha 1-antitryspsin deficiency (1), Fanconi anemia (1), Hunter syndrome (mild type) (1), chronic granulomatous disease (1), and purine nucleoside phosphorylase (PNP) deficiency (1).

Since Albert Gore, Jr., introduced his bill to establish a President's Commission on the Human Applications of Genetic Engineering in April 1983, there have been no major initiatives by the United States Congress to regulate human gene therapy. The Congress and the executive branch, as well, have seemed content with the national public review process for gene therapy as it has been carried out by the Human Gene Therapy Subcommittee (through 1991) and by the NIH Recombinant DNA Advisory Committee. The fact that the Food and Drug Administration has strengthened its capability to perform in-house, confidential reviews of gene therapy studies also provides reassurance to public policymakers.[31]

Numerous countries have established RAC-like committees to provide national review for gene therapy protocols. These countries include the United Kingdom, France, Canada, the Netherlands, Italy, and Japan. A major difference between most of the other committees and the RAC is that they meet in private and only announce their conclusions in public.

As gene therapy moves into the second half of its first clinical decade, somatic cell gene therapy is widely accepted in principle by opinion leaders and public policymakers. (For a listing of 28 policy statements on human genetic intervention by government committees, professional committees, and religious leaders, see Chapter 2.) There are initial promising results in a handful of gene therapy studies, and both newer biotechnology companies and more established pharmaceutical companies are increasingly interested in this field. We hope that the review process for gene therapy will continue to inform the general public about the field and will continue to protect potential recipients of gene therapy from undue risk of harm. We also hope that the countless hours invested in this research by hundreds of investigators and patients will bear fruit, and that gene therapy will one day play a central role in the conquest of human disease.

Notes

1. See, for example, Gordon Wolstenholme, ed., *Man and His Future* (London: J. & A. Churchill, 1963); Paul Ramsey, "Moral and Religious Aspects of Genetic Control," in John D. Roslansky, ed., *Genetics and the Future of Man* (Amsterdam: North-Holland Publishing Company, 1966), pp. 107–169; and Karl Rahner, "The Experiment with Man: Theological Observations on Man's Self-Manipulation," in his *Theological Investigations*, Vol. IX, translated by Graham Harrison (New York: Herder and Herder, 1972), 205–224 (Rahner's essay was published in German in 1966).

2. *Science* 157(3789): 633; 11 August 1967.

3. *Science* 158(3799): 313; 20 October 1967.

4. United States, Congress, Senate, Committee on Government Operations, Subcommittee on Government Research, *National Commission on Health Science and Society*, Hearings on S.J. Res. 145, 90th Congress, 2d Session, March 7–April 2, 1968 (Washington, DC: U.S. Government Printing Office, 1968), p. 448.

5. *United States Statutes at Large* 86:136–139 (enacted May 16, 1972).

6. *Genetic Screening: Programs, Principles, and Research* (Washington, DC: National Academy of Sciences, 1975).

7. David A. Jackson and Stephen P. Stich, *The Recombinant DNA Debate* (Englewood Cliffs, NJ: Prentice-Hall, 1979); Sheldon Krimsky, *Genetic Alchemy: The Social History of Recombinant DNA* (Cambridge, MA: MIT Press, 1982); United States, Congress, Congressional Research Service, Science Policy Research Division, *Genetic Engineering, Human Genetics, and Cell Biology: Evolution of Technological Issues—Biotechnology*, Supplemental Report III (Washington, DC: U.S. Government Printing Office, August 1980). The last-named report was prepared for the Subcommittee on Science, Research and Technology of the House Committtee on Science and Technology.

8. *U.S. Reports*, 447: 303–322 (decided June 16, 1980).

9. United States, President's Commission for the Study of Ethical Problems in Medicine and Biomedical and Behavioral Research, *Splicing Life: A Report on the Social and Ethical Issues of Genetic Engineering with Human Beings* (Washington, DC: The Commission, November 1982), pp. 95–96.

10. Ibid., p. 8.

11. Paul Jacobs, "Pioneer Genetic Implants Revealed," *Los Angeles Times*, October 8, 1980, pp. 1, 26.

12. Larry Thompson, *Correcting the Code: Inventing the Genetic Cure for the Human Body* (New York: Simon and Schuster, 1994), Chapter 7.

13. *New England Journal of Medicine* 303(22): 1293–1297; 27 November 1980.

14. *New England Journal of Medicine* 303(22): 1297–1300; 27 November 1980.

15. Testimony of Bernard Talbot, in United States, Congress, House, Committee on Science and Technology, Subcommittee on Investigations and Oversight, *Human Genetic Engineering*, Hearings, 97th Congress, 2d Session, November 16–18, 1982 (Washington, DC: U.S. Government Printing Office, 1982), pp. 543–545.

16. Council of Europe, Parliamentary Assembly, "Motion for a Recommendation on Protection of Humanity against Genetic Engineering and Artifiicial Fertilization," Document 4493, 31 January 1980, in *Documents, Working Papers*, 31st Ordinary Session, Third Part, January 28–February 1980, Vol. IX (Strasbourg: The Council, 1980).

17. Council of Europe, Parliamentary Assembly, *Genetic Engineering: Risks and Chances for Human Rights: Verbatim Report* (Strasbourg: The Council, 1981 [1982]).

18. Council of Europe, Parliamentary Assembly, "Report on Genetic Engineering," Document 4832, 18 January 1982, in *Documents, Working Papers*, 33rd Session, Third Part, January 25–29, Volume VII (Strasbourg: the Council, 1982).

19. Council of Europe, Parliamentary Assembly, *Texts Adopted by the Assembly*, 33rd Ordinary Session, Third Part, January 25–29 (Strasbourg: The Council, 1982).

20. Ibid.

21. U.S., President's Commission (note 9).

22. U.S., Congress, House, *Human Genetic Engineering* (note 15), p. 453.

23. U.S., Congress, House, "A Bill to Establish the President's Commission on the Human Applications of Genetic Engineering." H.R. 2788, 98th Congress, 1st Session, 27 April 1983.

24. U.S., President's Commission (note 9), pp. 84–87.

25. For another account and a chronology of the events in the next several paragraphs, see LeRoy Walters, "Human Gene Therapy: Ethics and Public Policy," *Human Gene Therapy* 2(2): 116–117, 119–120; Summer 1991.

26. National Institutes of Health, Recombinant DNA Advisory Committee, "Recombinant DNA Research: Request for Public Comment on 'Points to Consider in the Design and Submission of Human Somatic-Cell Gene Therapy Protocols,'" *Federal Register* 50(14): 2940–2945; 22 January 1985.

27. National Institutes of Health, Recombinant DNA Advisory Committee, "Recombinant DNA Molecules Research, Proposed Actions Under the Guidelines: Notice," *Federal Register* 50(160): 33462–33467; 19 August 1985.

28. For the full text of the most recent version of the "Points to Consider," see Appendix D.

29. For a detailed discussion of these and other ethical principles, see Tom L. Beauchamp and James F. Childress, *Principles of Biomedical Ethics* (4th ed.; New York: Oxford University Press, 1994).

30. Steven A. Rosenberg et al., "Gene Transfer Into Humans—Immunotherapy of Patients With Advanced Melanoma, Using Tumor-Infiltrating Lymphocytes Modified by Retroviral Gene Transduction," *New England Journal of Medicine* 323(9): 570–578; 30 August 1990.

31. David A. Kessler et al., "Regulation of Somatic-Cell Therapy and Gene Therapy by the Food and Drug Administration," *New England Journal of Medicine* 329(16): 1169–1173; 14 October 1993.

Appendix A:
Further Information
on Mitosis and Meiosis

Mitosis

There are two kinds of cell divisions: mitosis and meiosis. Mitotic division is the process whereby one cell divides to give rise to two that are genetically identical to the parent. It is mitosis that allows a single fertilized oocyte to give rise to a complete human being with its estimated 10^{14} cells, all (with a few exceptions) genetically identical to the original single cell. In mitosis, each daughter cell must receive the complete chromosome complement of 46 chromosomes.

Mitosis itself, the process of nuclear division, takes only a short time. However, it is part of a carefully programmed process, diagrammed in Figure A-1, called the cell cycle. Just after division, the cell that is destined to divide again enters a stage called G1 whereas one that will not enters a resting phase called G0. A cell in G1 next moves into S phase, during which time DNA replication occurs, by the semiconservative mechanism . . . wherein each DNA strand serves as a template for its own replication. The result is that each of the 46 chromosomes is duplicated into "sister chromatids," held together by a central constriction called the centromere. At the end of S phase, another gap phase (G2) begins, which then leads into actual mitosis (M).

In mitosis (Fig. A-2) the sister chromatids and the centromere become clearly visible and line up along the plane of eventual cleavage. The centromeres of all

Source: Thomas D. Gelehrter and Francis S. Collins, *Principles of Medical Genetics* (Baltimore: Williams & Wilkins, 1990), pp. 19–21. Reprinted by permission of the publisher.

155

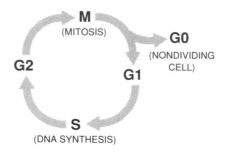

Figure A–1. The cell cycle.

46 chromosomes then divide, so that one sister chromatid from each ends up in the daughter cell, completing the cell cycle.

Meiosis and Gametogenesis

Meiosis, the variety of cell division that is used to generate the male and female gametes (sperm and oocytes, respectively), is different in crucial ways from mitosis. A little reflection suggests this must be so: if sperm and egg cells contained the full complement ("diploid") set of 46 chromosomes, the fertilized oocyte would have 92 chromosomes, including three X's and a Y!

Meiosis, the special reduction process that is carried out in gametogenesis to generate sperm and egg cells, each bearing 23 chromosomes (the "haploid" state), is diagrammed in Figure A-3. There are actually two divisions, meiosis I and meiosis II. In meiosis I, each chromosome replicates into sister chromatids, just as in mitosis. Unlike mitosis, however, the homologous chromosomes then align in pairs (a process called synapsis) and separate to *opposite* poles, with their sister chromatids still together. In meiosis II, the sister chromatids then separate, resulting in 23 chromosomes per gamete.

Crossing Over

An extremely important feature of meiosis I is that during synapsis, when homologous chromosomes are paired together, crossovers occur (Fig. A-4). The practical result of this is that the chromosome retained in a gamete at the end of meiosis may be a patchwork of *both* homologous parental chromosomes. Genes that are close together on a chromosome, however (such as A and B in Figure A-4), are likely to be passed along together, whereas a crossover (or "recombination") is more likely to occur between genes that are far apart on a chromosome. On the average, about 30–40 crossovers (or 1–2 per chromosome) occur during a meiotic division.

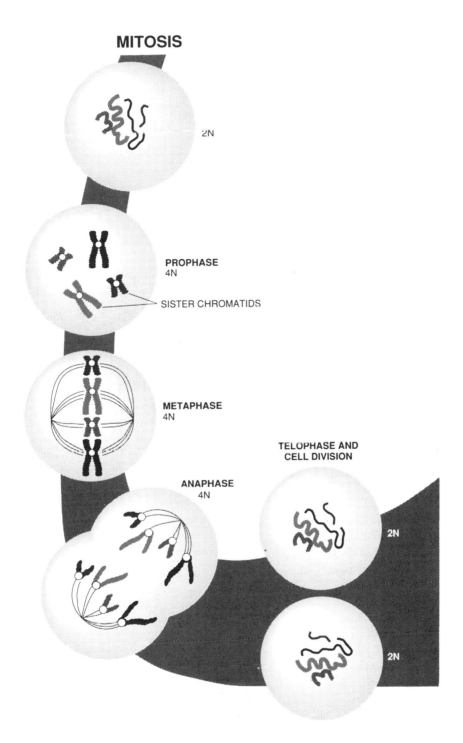

Figure A–2. Mitosis. For simplicity only four chromosomes, consisting of two pairs of autosomes are shown. The "ploidy" of the cell is shown at each stage: 2N represents the diploid state. After formation of sister chromatids but before cell division, the cell contains an amount of DNA corresponding to 4N.

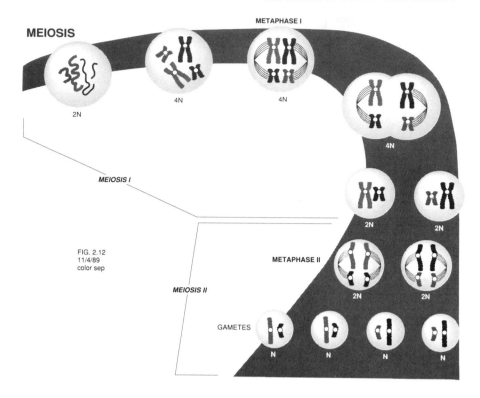

Figure A–3. Meiosis. Again, only two pairs of autosomes are shown. Note that after meiosis I each cell only retains *one* of the homologous pair. Meiosis II then leads to sister chromatid separation. For simplicity, no crossing over is shown.

Besides increasing enormously the potential genetic diversity of gametes, crossing over provides a quantitative estimate of the distance separating two genes on the same chromosome (called "syntenic" genes). . . . [T]his has provided a powerful means of mapping genes.

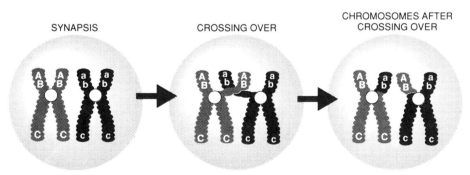

Figure A–4. Crossing over in meiosis I.

Appendix B:
Background Information
on Mendelian Inheritance

Chromosomes and Inheritance

Higher organisms package their DNA into segments called chromosomes. Each chromosome is composed of one very long stretch of DNA that is bound to various proteins and other molecules. There are two copies of each of 22 chromosomes in the cells of a human. In addition, there are two sex chromosomes. Females have two "X" chromosomes and males have one "X" and one "Y." In normal human cells, therefore, there are 46 chromosomes: 2 sex chromosomes and 2 copies of each of 22 other chromosomes (these non-sex chromosomes are called **autosomes**).

The 46 discrete aggregates of DNA and attached protein that comprise the chromosomes are maintained inside the nucleus of somatic cells. In germ cells, in contrast, a specialized phenomenon called meiosis takes place. Cells divide so as to leave only 23 chromosomes in a sperm cell or ovum: one sex chromosome (either an "X" or a "Y") and *one* copy of each of the autosomes. All ova contain an "X" and 22 autosomes, because they derive from female cells that contain two "X" chromosomes. Sperm are divided into two groups; half have an "X" and 22 autosomes and the other half have a "Y" plus 22 autosomes.

During the process of fertilization, a sperm joins with an ovum to restore the chromosome number to 46. If the sperm contains an "X" chromosome then a female is produced, and if it contains a "Y" then a male results.

Source: United States, Congress, Office of Technology Assessment, *Human Gene Therapy: Background Paper* (Washington, DC: OTA, December 1984), pp. 13–16.

Single Gene, Multigene, and Environmentally Modified Traits

Diseases that might be treated by gene therapy will, at least in the foreseeable future, be exclusively those caused by mutations in a single gene. Such diseases are called single gene defects, and contrast with diseases and traits influenced by several genes or environmental factors. Genes can cause disease through several mechanisms. Most human diseases have a genetic component inherited by the individual and an environmental component that comes from outside the individual. The relative importance of genetic and environmental influences varies in both patients and diseases. Some medical conditions, such as automobile accidents or war wounds, may have large environmental and very small genetic contributions. Most diseases have a mixture of genetic and environmental contributions (Harsanyi, 1981). In several disorders, such as Huntington or Tay-Sachs diseases, the influence of a single gene is so large that the disorders are called genetic diseases.

Single Gene Traits, or Mendelian Traits

When traits or diseases are primarily determined by a single gene, they obey the relatively simple laws of inheritance first specified by Gregor Mendel, a monk who lived in the last century and whose interests in agriculture led him to discover several genetic phenomena in plants. The same patterns of inheritance that Mendel first described in plants, noted below, are also found in several human diseases, and thus indicate that the cause of the disease is genetic.

At the turn of the century, a British physician and scientist, Archibald Garrod, first introduced the idea that some diseases that followed definite inheritance patterns might be caused by "inborn errors of metbolism" (Stanbury, 1983; Kevles, 1984). He postulated that some diseases were due to biochemical errors. He further speculated that such biochemical defects might be caused by genetic abnormalities that obey Mendel's laws. Several decades later, biochemical errors were, for first time, traced to specific enzymes. These discoveries confirmed Garrod's hypothesis. Other diseases were traced to molecular defects in non-enzyme proteins; the first "molecular disease" described was sickle cell anemia, in which an abnormal hemoglobin protein was found (Pauling, 1949). Research over the past three decades has revealed more and more genetic diseases, and greater understanding of many of them.

Many genetic diseases are due to changes in just a single gene, such as ADA and PNP deficiencies. More than two hundred specific enzyme defects cause known human clinical syndromes, and over a hundred other genetic diseases have been biochemically characterized (Stanbury, 1983). Prominent disorders such as sickle cell anemia, familial hypercholesterolemia, polycystic kidney disease, Huntington disease, neurofibromatosis, Duchenne muscular dystrophy, cystic fibrosis, achondroplasia, hemophilia, and many others are examples of single gene disorders. Many common adult disorders, usually excluded from pediatric statistics on genetic disease prevalence, such as Alzheimer disease and hemochromatosis, have forms strongly influenced by genetics (Breitner, 1984; Cook, 1979, 1981; Folstein, 1981; Cartwright, 1978, Dadone, 1982; Skolnick, 1982; Kravitz, 1979). Single gene defects affect 1 to 2 percent of newborns (Lubs, 1977), and addition of adult genetic diseases would significantly increase the estimated prevalence and cost of genetic disease.

Even diseases or traits that are due to a single gene vary widely in severity, depending on environmental factors and other genes; the extent to which patients have signs and symptoms of a genetic disease is called "expressivity." Diseases can also be variably expressed in populations, affecting some people and not others who carry the gene. This is described as "penetrance." Complete penetrance indicates that all who have the defective gene also have the disease, while incomplete penetrance means that some people have the gene but not the disease.

Single gene traits can be classified by how they are inherited. They can be recessive, dominant, or X-linked.

Recessive disorders. Recessive diseases occur when one receives a defective gene from both parents (Fig. B-1). Diseases due to dysfunctional gene pairs are usually due to protein abnormalities that cause a biochemical imbalance. Sickle cell disease and thalassemia affect globin, the protein part of hemoglobin, which transports oxygen through the blood to body tissues. Other recessive disorders, such as Tay-Sachs disease, ADA and PNP deficiencies, and phenylketonuria (PKU), affect enzymes whose absence or dysfunction adversely affects cellular metabolism. Most of the relatively well understood genetic diseases are recessive disorders that can be traced to specific defects in enzymes. However, the specific molecular defect underlying many recessive diseases, including at least one common one—cystic fibrosis—is not known.

Dominant disorders. Dominant disorders occur when offspring receive a defective gene from *either* parent, and having just one such gene leads to expression of the disease (Fig. B-2). In some cases the defect is known, such as some types of porphyria, in which enzyme deficiencies lead to abnormal disruption of biochemical pathways that produce and degrade heme—the non-protein part of hemoglobin found in red blood cells. In most dominant disorders, however, the biochemical nature of the derangement is not known; the molecular defect in dominant disorders is, in general, less well established than for recessive ones.

X-linked disorders. X-linked disorders are carried on the "X" chromosome. (Fig. B-3). X-linked diseases usually affect boys because males have only one copy of the "X" chromosome: there is no set of genes on a second "X" chromosome to balance the effects of a defective copy of the gene. The inheritance pat-

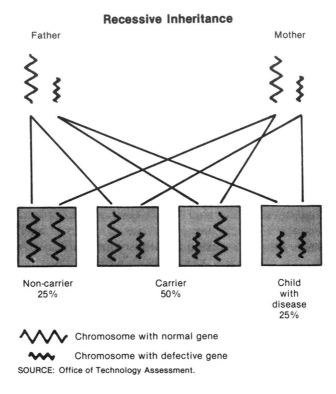

Recessive Inheritance

Father   Mother

Non-carrier   Carrier   Child
25%   50%   with
                                      disease
                                      25%

〰〰 Chromosome with normal gene
〰 Chromosome with defective gene
SOURCE: Office of Technology Assessment.

Figure B–1. Recessive inheritance.

tern of X-linked disorders is distinctive: sons inherit the traits only from their mothers, because a son always derives his "X" from his mother and his "Y" from his father. Daughters can get a defective gene from either parent, but do not usually have the disease unless they get the abnormal gene from *both* parents. X-linked traits thus act like dominant traits inherited only from the mother in boys, and are usually recessive in girls. Examples of X-linked disease traits are hemophilia, Duchenne muscular dystrophy, and Lesch-Nyhan syndrome.

There are apparently few traits, and no known diseases, that are carried in genes located on the "Y" chromosome, and expressed only in males.

Single gene defects are, in general, the best understood of genetic diseases; the early instances of human gene therapy will be done to correct the effects of single mutant genes.

Multigene Traits

There are certain body characteristics and other traits that accrue from the interactions of several genes. Eye and hair color, for example, are traits that are speci-

Dominant Inheritance

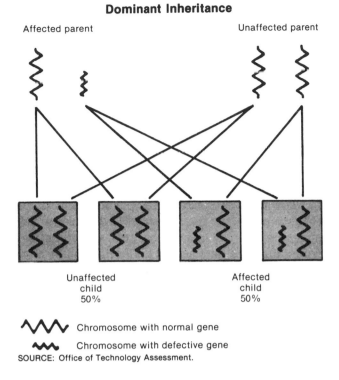

Figure B–2. Dominant inheritance.

fied by genes, but do not obey simple Mendelian patterns of inheritance because many genes are involved. Similarly, there are genetic diseases caused by interactions of multiple genes that are minimally affected by environmental influences. Such disorders are termed polygenic or multigenic.

Environmentally Modified Traits

The vast majority of characteristics that define individuals are determined by a combination of genetic predisposition and interaction with the environment. Height, for example, though determined genetically to a significant extent, is also influenced by nutrition and other factors. Likewise, many diseases derive from interactions of genes and the environment in which both components contribute significantly to the disease process.

The type of diabetes mellitus that occurs in younger people, for example, is now believed to be caused by a special susceptibility of insulin-secreting cells to certain viral infections or other environmental insults. The clinical disorder is thus caused by an environmental agent acting in concert with genetic characteristics.

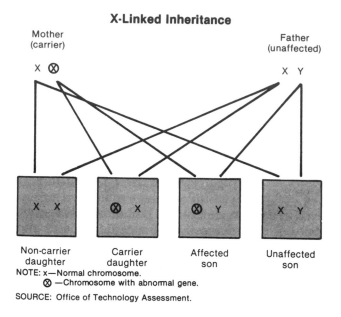

Figure B–3. X-linked inheritance.

Most common diseases, including cardiovascular diseases, cancer, and many drug reactions appear to involve multiple genes as well as environmental influences.

Most complex human traits, including physical and intellectual capacities, are also multigenic and environmentally influenced. The controversies that have raged in the psychological literature over the genetic and racial components of intelligence center on the relative importance of genetic and environmental contributions, including nutrition, health care, cultural background, and socioeconomic status. There is little doubt that genetics and environment interact, but there is vigorous contention about which factor predominates and how public policy should respond to differences in complex traits such as intelligence.

References

J. C. S. Breitner and M. F. Folstein, "Familial Alzheimer Dementia: A Prevalent Disorder With Specific Clinical Features," *Psychological Medicine* 14:63–80; 1984.

G. E. Cartwright, M. Skolnick, D. B. Amos, et al., "Inheritance of Hemochromatosis: Linkage to HLA," *Transactions of the Association of American Physicians* 16:273–281; 1978.

R. H. Cook, B. Ward, and J. H. Austin, "Studies in Aging of the Brain, IV. Familial Alzheimer Disease: Relation to Transmissible Dementia, Aneuploidy, and Microtubular Defects," *Neurology* 29:1402–1412; 1979.

R. H. Cook, S. A. Schneck, and D. B. Clark, "Twins With Alzheimer's Disease," *Archives of Neurology* 38:300–301; 1981.

M. M. Dadone, J. P. Kushner, C. Q. Edwards, et al., "Hereditary Hemochromatosis," *American Journal of Clinical Pathology* 78:196–207; 1982.

M. F. Folstein and J. C. S. Breitner, "Language Disorder Predicts Familial Alzheimer's Disease," *Johns Hopkins Medical Journal* 149:145–147; 1981.

Z. Harsanyi and R. Hutton, *Genetic Prophecy: Beyond the Double Helix* (New York: Rawson, Wade, 1981).

D. J. Kevles, "Annals of Eugenics: A Secular Faith," series of four articles appearing in the *The New Yorker*, Oct. 8, 1984, pp. 51ff.; Oct. 15, 1984, pp. 52ff.; Oct. 22, 1984, pp. 92ff.; Oct. 29, 1984, pp. 51ff.

K. Kravitz, M. Skolnick, C. Cannings, et al.,"Genetic Linkage Between Hereditary Hemochromatosis and HLA," *American Journal of Human Genetics* 31:601–619; 1979.

H. A. Lubs, "Frequency of Genetic Disease," in Lubs, H. A., and de la Cruz, F., *Genetic Counseling* (New York: Raven, 1977), pp. 1–16.

L. Pauling, H. A. Itano, S. J. Singer, and I. C. Wells, "Sickle Cell Anemia: A Molecular Disease," *Science* 110:543–548; 1949.

M. H. Skolnick, Testimony at a Hearing before the Subcommittee on Investigations and Oversight of the Committee on Science and Technology, U.S. House of Representatives, Nov. 16–18, 1982. Reprinted in *Human Genetic Engineering*, U.S. Government Printing Office, Committee Print No. 170, 1983; pp. 242–274.

J. B. Stanbury, J. B. Wyngaarden, D. S. Fredrickson, J. L. Goldstein, and M. S. Brown, "Inborn Errors of Metabolism," *The Metabolic Basis of Inherited Disease*, ch. 1, 5th ed. (New York: McGraw-Hill, 1983).

Appendix C:
Additional Methods for
Delivering Genes to Cells

Delivery in Vitro

DNA Viruses

Although retroviruses provide the most efficient vehicle for delivering genes to cells in vitro, researchers have devised several other methods for delivering genes into cells in vitro, some of which are useful in circumstances where transduction by disabled retroviruses is not practical.

Viruses that have DNA rather than RNA in their cores can be useful vectors. For example, adeno-associated viruses (AAV)—nonpathogenic viruses that can integrate into host cell genomes—have certain worthwhile characteristics, such as the ability to reach high concentrations in solution, which are not found in retroviruses.[1] Other DNA viruses, such as herpes viruses, which do not integrate into host chromosomes but remain stable and separate in host cells, have also been exploited as delivery vehicles. Herpes viruses have large genomes and a high capacity for incorporating large foreign sequences, making them suitable vectors for the delivery of large genes into host cells. Nonintegrating vectors have the advantage of being able to survive in nonreplicating cells, in contrast to integrating retroviruses, which can only transfer genes into replicating cells because they use the cells' replication machinery for integration.[2]

Naked DNA

Several of these methods, collectively called *transfection*, involve the delivery of naked DNA (without a protein envelope) into cells in vitro.[3] For example, naked

DNA can be physically injected into cells, using very fine micropipettes and a machine that is so sensitive that it sits on a cushion of air to prevent random vibrations of the building in which it sits from jarring its delicate instruments. This procedure, known as *microinjection*, is carried out and viewed under the lens of the machine's microscope. Microinjection is an efficient delivery method but requires the investment of too much time, energy, and resources per cell to be practical for transfecting more than a small number of cells.[4]

Another method of transfection involves adding calcium phosphate, coprecipitated with DNA, to cells in vitro. *Calcium phosphate coprecipitation* allows cells to take up DNA; how this occurs is poorly understood.[5] Although this method is inefficient (only about 10% of the exposed cells successfully acquire the DNA), it is useful for treating large populations of cells at one time.[6]

A third method of transfection is *electroporation*, in which cells are exposed to rapid pulses of high voltage current that create reparable holes in the cell membranes and cause the cells to take up DNA from the surrounding medium.[7] Like calcium phosphate coprecipitation, electroporation is relatively inefficient.

Artificial membrane sacs, called *liposomes*, provide a fourth method of transfection. Researchers can fill liposome sacs with DNA and deliver that DNA into human cells by fusing the liposomes with the recipient cells.[8]

Most of these methods for transfecting cells with naked DNA are inefficient—able to deliver DNA to only a fraction of the exposed cells. Accordingly, they are most often used in conjunction with methods for recognizing and selecting the fraction of cells that do take up DNA.

Delivery in Vivo

The transduction and transfection methods described allow the introduction of genes into cells in vitro. In vitro delivery is useful for gene therapy if the cells to which one desires to add DNA, like T cells, can be removed from the body of the patient receiving treatment. In most cases, it is not practical or possible to remove target cells from patients' bodies. For instance, it is not realistic to propose the removal of target cells for gene therapy of a genetic brain disease or for a disease that affects many different cell types throughout a patient's body. Even when removal of target cells is possible, in vitro gene delivery may be invasive and impractical, requiring specialists and hospitalization for the gene therapy's success.

Delivering genes to cells in vivo ("within the living organism")[9] offers the potential to treat a broader range of diseases and may be a less invasive form of treatment. Researchers are contemplating several potential methods for in vivo gene delivery. One approach, described in chapter 2 in the context of a genetic disease called familial hypercholesterolemia, involves the creation of recombinant viral packages that will deliver genes in vivo.[10] A risk of this technique is the possibility that, like most viruses, the recombinant viral packages will transduce many different cell types.[11] (The dangers of transmitting genes into cells where they are not needed or where they could be deleterious are addressed in chapter 2.) Hence, researchers are developing recombinant viruses ensheathed in protein coats that recognize specific cell types.

A different strategy involves the introduction of genes directly into a target organ. Both naked DNA and DNA complexed with various other substances have been used with some success for direct in vivo delivery of genes.[12] For example, one research team reported that by injecting "pure RNA and DNA directly into mouse skeletal muscle," it obtained "significant expression" of the included genes within the muscle cells.[13]

Cell Grafting

A third approach to delivering genes involves a combination of in vitro and in vivo gene delivery procedures. This method, called *cell grafting*, entails the transfer of genes into cells that have been removed and which can, upon their return to the body, metabolically cooperate with nonremovable cells. The removable cells are harvested, cultured, and subjected to gene transfer using one of the many methods developed for transferring genes into cells in vitro. When these corrected cells are replaced into a living organism, they produce the desired gene products and transmit them to the cells where they are needed.

This approach may prove fruitful for the treatment of Parkinson disease.[14] Parkinson's is a degenerative neurological disorder resulting from the progressive loss of a specific class of cells, the neurons that produce dopamine in the part of the brain known as the *substantia nigra*. Patients who suffer from Parkinson disease have slowly progressing tremors, muscle stiffness, and balance and coordination problems. These symptoms can be ameliorated with a drug known as L-*dopa*, which is converted to dopamine by the patients' own bodies. L-*dopa* therapy can lose efficacy over time, however, and can cause serious side effects. Accordingly, researchers are looking for alternative treatments for this disease, which affects about 200,000 Americans annually.

Using animal models of Parkinson disease, researchers have demonstrated that recovery from symptoms can be achieved by transplanting genetically modified cells into the brains of affected animals. Researchers have genetically modified skin fibroblasts so that they express tyrosine hydroxylase (TH), which allows them to produce and release L-dopa. The researchers have then implanted these L-dopa producing cells in the brains of rats suffering from an animal version of Parkinson disease. This strategy has resulted in the reduction of the rats' behavioral abnormalities.[15] Similar experiments using genetically modified fibroblasts or fetal cells have prevented the deterioration or caused the regeneration of the critical neurons in animal models of Parkinson's disease.[16] In addition, researchers have implanted genetically modified muscle cells into rat brains and thereby reduced abnormal behavior in the rat model of Parkinson's disease.[17] In all of these experiments, researchers are relying on the ability of the implanted cells to cooperate with neuronal cells that are unable to produce dopamine in the affected animals.[18]

H. E. Gruber and his colleagues are working on a treatment for the tragic disease Lesch-Nyhan syndrome. The absence of a functioning version of an enzyme called HPRT causes neural dysfunction, mental retardation, spasticity, and a characteristic behavior of self-mutilation in Lesch-Nyhan syndrome patients.[19] Gruber's team and others have demonstrated that one type of cell that contains functioning HPRT can cooperate with another type of cell in which the HPRT gene is defective. Gruber and his colleagues postulate that, using cell grafting, they might employ metabolic cooperation to prevent nonremovable mutant neuronal cells in Lesch-Nyhan patients from functioning aberrantly.[20]

One futuristic gene delivery system, a type of cell grafting, uses artificial-organ-like structures to place functioning genes into the body. These *organoids* or *neo-organs* theoretically would be implanted into human patients' abdominal cavities, where they would deliver desired gene products into the circulation. For example, Philippe Moullier and colleagues in France have prepared lattices made of cells containing a retroviral vector carrying the human B-glucuronidase gene, plus collagen and polytetrafluoroethylene (PTFE) fibers coated with heparin and basic fibroblast growth factor (BFGF). They then implanted these structures into the peritoneal cavities of dogs. Neo-organs developed rapidly and provided an environment which allowed the cells containing the retroviral vectors to survive and to produce recombinant enzyme that reached distant organs in the dogs' bodies.[21] In parallel fashion, researchers at the Massachusetts Institute of Technology and at the University of Alabama have also explored artificial systems for delivering genes and their products to patients.[22]

Notes

1. Theodore Friedmann, "Progress Toward Human Gene Therapy," *Science* 244(4910): 1277; 16 June 1989.

2. Ibid.

3. Maxine Singer and Paul Berg, *Genes and Genomes: A Changing Perspective* (Mill Valley, CA: University Science Books, 1991), p. 299; Robert C. King and William D. Stansfield, *A Dictionary of Genetics* (4th ed.; New York: Oxford University Press, 1990), pp. 316–317.

4. Singer and Berg (note 3).

5. Ibid.

6. Ibid.

7. Ibid.; Friedmann op. cit., p. 1275.

8. King and Stansfield, op. cit., p. 181; Theodore Friedmann, *Gene Therapy: Fact and Fiction in Biology's New Approaches to Disease* (Cold Spring Harbor, NY: Banbury Center, Cold Spring Harbor Laboratory, 1983), p. 39.

9. King and Stansfield, op. cit., p. 167.

10. See also United States, President's Commission for the Study of Ethical Problems in Medicine and Biomedical and Behavioral Research, *Splicing Life: A Report on the Social and Ethical Issues of Genetic Engineering with Human Beings* (Washington, DC: the Commission, November 1982), p. 43.

11. Frank Costantini, Gene Therapy Lecture for Medical Genetics 1015, Columbia University (March 15, 1983).

12. Friedmann, "Progress," p. 1279.

13. Jon A. Wolff et al., "Direct Gene Transfer into Mouse Muscle in Vivo," *Science* 247(4949, Part 1): 1465–1468; 23 March 1990.

14. See Leon Jaroff, "Giant Step for Gene Therapy," *Time*, September 24, 1990, p. 76.

15. Jon A. Wolff et al., "Grafting Fibroblasts Genetically Modified to Produce L-Dopa in a Rat Model of Parkinson Disease," *Proceedings of the National Academy of Sciences* 86(22): 9011–9014; November 1989.

16. David M. Frim et al., "Implanted Fibroblasts Genetically Engineered to Produce Brain-Derived Neurotrophic Factor Prevent 1-Methyl-4-Phenylpyridinium Toxicity to Dopaminergic Neurons in the Rat," *Proceedings of the National Academy of Sciences* 91(11): 5104–5108; 24 May 1994; and Shu Ming Zhu, "Implantation of Genetically Modified Mesencephalic Fetal Cells into the Rat Striatum," *Brain Research Bulletin* 29(1): 81–93; July 1992.

17. Shoushu Jiao, "Long-Term Correction of Rat Model of Parkinson's Disease by Gene Therapy," *Nature* 362(6419): 450–453; 1 April 1993.

18. Other researchers have experimented with an alternative approach to Parkinson disease, injecting vectors expressing TH directly into rodent brain cells in vivo. See Matthew J. During et al., "Long-Term Behavioral Recovery in Parkinsonian Rats by HSV Vector Expressing Tyrosine Hydroxylase," *Science* 266(5189): 1399–1403; 25 November 1994; and Michael G. Kaplitt et al., "Long-Term Gene Expression and Phenotypic Correction Using Adeno-Associated Virus Vectors in the Mammalian Brain," *Nature Genetics* 8(2): 148–154; October 1994.

19. David W. Melton, "HPRT Gene Organization and Expression," *Oxford Surveys on Eukaryotic Genes* 4: 34–76; 1987; David Suzuki and Peter Knudtson, *Genethics: The Clash Between the New Genetics and Human Values* (Cambridge, MA: Harvard University Press, 1989), p. 168.

20. H. E. Gruber et al., "Glial Cells Metabolically Cooperate: A Potential Requirement for Gene Replacement Therapy," *Proceedings of the National Academy of Sciences* 82(19): 6662–6666; October 1985; Friedmann, "Progress" (note 1), p. 1278. See also Jon A. Wolff and Theodore Friedmann, "Approaches to Gene Therapy in Disorders of Purine Metabolism," *Rheumatic Disease Clinics of North America* 14(2): 459–477; August 1988.

21. Philippe Moullier et al., "Long-Term Delivery of a Lysosomal Enzyme by Genetically Modified Fibroblasts in Dogs," *Nature Medicine* 1(4): 353–357; April 1995.

22. Beverly Merz, "Gene Therapy Enters 'Second Generation,'" *American Medical News*, December 22/29, 1989, pp. 3, 11.

Appendix D:
The "Points to Consider" Developed by the NIH Recombinant DNA Advisory Committee

Appendix M. The Points to Consider in the Design and Submission of Protocols for the Transfer of Recombinant DNA Molecules into the Genome of One or More Human Subjects (Points to Consider)

Appendix M applies to research conducted at or sponsored by an institution that receives any support for recombinant DNA research from the NIH. Researchers not covered by the *NIH Guidelines* are encouraged to use Appendix M.

The acceptability of human somatic cell gene therapy has been addressed in several public documents as well as in numerous academic studies. In November 1982, The President's Commission for the Study of Ethical Problems in Medicine and Biomedical and Behavioral Research published a report, *Splicing Life*, which resulted from a two-year process of public deliberation and hearings. Upon release of that report, a U.S. House of Representatives subcommittee held three days of public hearings with witnesses from a wide range of fields from the biomedical and social sciences to theology, philosophy, and law. In December 1984, the Office of Technology Assessment released a background paper, *Human Gene Therapy*, which concluded: "Civic, religious, scientific, and medical groups have all accepted, in principle, the appropriateness of gene therapy of somatic cells in humans for specific genetic diseases. Somatic cell gene therapy is seen as an extension of present methods of therapy that might be preferable to other tech-

Source: United States, National Institutes of Health, "Recombinant DNA Research: Actions under the Guidelines," *Federal Register* 60(81): 20731-20737; 27 April 1995.

171

nologies." In light of this public support, the Recombinant DNA Advisory Committee (RAC) is prepared to consider proposals for somatic cell gene transfer.

The RAC will not at present entertain proposals for germ line alterations but will consider proposals involving somatic cell gene transfer. The purpose of somatic cell gene therapy is to treat an individual patient, e.g., by inserting a properly functioning gene into the subject's somatic cells. Germ line alteration involves a specific attempt to introduce genetic changes into the germ (reproductive) cells of an individual, with the aim of changing the set of genes passed on to the individual's offspring.

In the interest of maximizing the resources of both the NIH and the Food and Drug Administration (FDA) and simplifying the method and period for review, research proposals involving the deliberate transfer of recombinant DNA or DNA or RNA derived from recombinant DNA into human subjects (human gene transfer) will be considered through a consolidated review process involving both the NIH and the FDA. Submission of human gene transfer proposals will be in the format described in Appendices M-I through M-V of the *Points to Consider*. Investigators must simultaneously submit their human gene transfer proposal to both the NIH and the FDA in a single submission format. This format includes (but is not limited to) the documentation described in Appendices M-I through M-V of the *Points to Consider*. NIH/ORDA and the FDA will simultaneously evaluate the proposal regarding the necessity for RAC review.

Factors that may contribute to the necessity for RAC review include: (i) new vectors/new gene delivery systems, (ii) new diseases, (iii) unique applications of gene transfer, and (iv) other issues considered to require further public discussion. Among the experiments that may be considered exempt from RAC review are those determined by the NIH/ORDA and FDA not to represent possible risk to human health or the environment (see Appendix M-VII, *Categories of Human Gene Transfer Experiments that May Be Exempt from RAC Review*). Whenever possible, investigators will be notified within 15 working days following receipt of the submission whether RAC review will be required. In the event that NIH/ORDA and the FDA require RAC review of the submitted proposal, the documentation described in Appendices M-I through M-V of the *Points to Consider* will be forwarded to the RAC primary reviewers for evaluation. RAC meetings will be open to the public except where trade secrets and proprietary information are reviewed. The RAC and FDA prefer that information provided in response to Appendix M contain no proprietary data or trade secrets, enabling all aspects of the review to be open to the public. The RAC will recommend approval or disapproval of the reviewed proposal to the NIH Director. In the event that a proposal is contingently approved by the RAC, the RAC prefers that the conditions be satisfactorily met before the RAC's recommendation for approval is submitted to the NIH Director. The NIH Director's decision on the submitted proposal will be transmitted to the FDA Commissioner and considered as a *Major Action* by the NIH Director.

Public review of human gene transfer proposals will serve to inform the public about the technical aspects of the proposals as well as the meaning and significance of the research.

In its evaluation of human gene transfer proposals, the RAC, NIH/ORDA, and the FDA will consider whether the design of such experiments offers adequate assurance that their consequences will not go beyond their purpose, which is the same as the traditional purpose of clinical investigation, namely, to protect the health and well being of human subjects being treated while at the same time gathering generalizable knowledge. Two possible undesirable consequences of the transfer of recombinant DNA would be unintentional: (I) vertical transmission of genetic changes from an individual to his/her offspring, or (ii) horizontal transmission of viral infection to other persons with whom the individual comes in contact. Accordingly, Appendices M-I through M-V request information that will enable the RAC, NIH/ORDA, and the FDA to assess the possibility that the proposed experiment(s) will inadvertently affect reproductive cells or lead to infection of other people (e.g., medical personnel or relatives).

In recognition of the social concern that surrounds the subject of human gene transfer, the RAC, NIH/ORDA, and the FDA, will cooperate with other groups in assessing the possible long-term consequences of the proposal and related laboratory and animal experiments in order to define appropriate human applications of this emerging technology.

Appendix M will be considered for revisions as experience in evaluating proposals accumulates and as new scientific developments occur. This review will be carried out periodically as needed.

Submission Requirements—Human Gene Transfer Proposals

Investigators must simultaneously submit the following material to both: (1) the Office of Recombinant DNA Activities (ORDA), National Institutes of Health, Suite 323, 6006 Executive Boulevard, MSC 7052, Bethesda, Maryland 20892-7052, (301 496-9838 (see exemption in Appendix M-IX-A, *Footnotes of Appendix M*); and (2) the Division of Congressional and Public Affairs, Document Control Center, HFM-99, Center for Biologics Evaluation and Research, 1401 Rockville Pike, Rockville, Maryland 20852-1448. Proposals will be submitted in the following order: (1) scientific abstract—1 page; (2) non-technical abstract—1 page; (3) Institutional Biosafety Committee and Institutional Review Board approvals and their deliberations pertaining to your protocol (The IBC and IRB may, at their discretion, condition their approval on further specific deliberation by the RAC); (4) Responses to Appendix M-II, *Description of the Proposal*—5 pages; (5) protocol (as approved by the local Institutional Biosafety Committee and Institutional Review Board)—20 pages; (6) Informed Consent document— approved by the Institutional Review Board (see Appendix M-III, *Informed Consent*); (7) appendices (including tables, figures, and manuscripts); (8) curricula vitae—2 pages for each key professional person in biographical sketch format; and (9) three 3½ inch diskettes with the complete vector nucleotide sequence in ASCII format.

Appendix M-II. Description of the Proposal

Responses to this appendix should be provided in the form of either written answers or references to specific sections of the protocol or its appendices. Investigators should indicate the points that are not applicable with a brief explanation. Investigators submitting proposals that employ the same vector systems may refer to preceding documents relating to the vector sequence without having to rewrite such material.

II-A. Objectives and Rationale of the Proposed Research

State concisely the overall objectives and rationale of the proposed study. Provide information on the specific points that relate to whichever type of research is being proposed.

II-A-1. Use of Recombinant DNA for Therapeutic Purposes

For research in which recombinant DNA is transferred in order to treat a disease or disorder (e.g., genetic diseases, cancer, and metabolic diseases), the following questions should be addressed:

II-A-1-a. Why is the disease selected for treatment by means of gene therapy a good candidate for such treatment?

II-A-1-b. Describe the natural history and range of expression of the disease selected for treatment. What objective and/or quantitative measures of disease activity are available? In your view, are the usual effects of the disease predictable enough to allow for meaningful assessment of the results of gene therapy?

II-A-1-c. Is the protocol designed to prevent all manifestations of the disease, to halt the progression of the disease after symptoms have begun to appear, or to reverse manifestations of the disease in seriously ill victims?

II-A-1-d. What alternative therapies exist? In what groups of patients are these therapies effective? What are their relative advantages and disadvantages as compared with the proposed gene therapy?

II-A-2. Transfer of DNA for Other Purposes

II-A-2-a. Into what cells will the recombinant DNA be transferred? Why is the transfer of recombinant DNA necessary for the proposed research? What questions can be answered by using recombinant DNA?

II-A-2-b. What alternative methodologies exist? What are their relative advantages and disadvantages as compared to the use of recombinant DNA?

II-B. Research Design, Anticipated Risks, and Benefits

II-B-1. Structure and Characteristics of the Biological System

Provide a full description of the methods and reagents to be employed for gene delivery and the rationale for their use. The following are specific points to be addressed:

II-B-1-a. What is the structure of the cloned DNA that will be used?

II-B-1-a-(1). Describe the gene (genomic or cDNA), the bacterial plasmid or phage vector, and the delivery vector (if any). Provide complete nucleotide sequence analysis or a detailed restriction enzyme map of the total construct.

II B-1-a-(2). What regulatory elements does the construct contain (e.g., promoters, enhancers, polyadenylation sites, replication origins, etc.)? From what source are these elements derived? Summarize what is currently known about the regulatory character of each element.

II-B-1-a-(3). Describe the steps used to derive the DNA construct.

II-B-1-b. What is the structure of the material that will be administered to the patient?

II-B-1-b-(1). Describe the preparation, structure, and composition of the materials that will be given to the patient or used to treat the patient's cells: (I) If DNA, what is the purity (both in terms of being a single DNA species and in terms of other contaminants)? What tests have been used and what is the sensitivity of the tests? (ii) If a virus, how is it prepared from the DNA construct? In what cell is the virus grown (any special features)? What medium and serum are used? How is the virus purified? What is its structure and purity? What steps are being taken (and assays used with their sensitivity) to detect and elminate any contaminating materials (for example, VL30 RNA, other nucleic acids, or proteins) or contaminating viruses (both replication-competent or replication-defective) or other organisms in the cells or serum used for preparation of the virus stock including any contaminants that may have biological effects? (iii) If co-cultivation is employed, what kinds of cells are being used for co-cultivation? What steps are being taken (and assays used with their sensitivity) to detect and eliminate any contaminating materials? Specifically, what tests are being conducted to assess the material to be returned to the patient for the presence of live or killed donor cells or other non-vector materials (for example, VL30 sequences) originating from those cells? (iv) If methods other than those covered by Appendices M-II-B-1 through M-II-B-3, *Research Design, Anticipated Risks and Benefits*, are used to introduce new genetic information into target cells, what steps are being taken to detect and eliminate any contaminating materials? What are possible sources of contamination? What is the sensitivity of tests used to monitor contamination?

II-B-1-b-(2). Describe any other material to be used in preparation of the material to be administered to the patient. For example, if a viral vector is proposed, what is the nature of the helper virus or cell line? If carrier particles are to be used, what is the nature of these?

II-B-2. Preclinical Studies, Including Risk-Assessment Studies

Provide results that demonstrate the safety, efficacy, and feasibility of the proposed procedures using animal and/or cell culture model systems, and explain why the model(s) chosen is/are most appropriate.

II-B-2-a. Delivery System

II-B-2-a-(1). What cells are the intended target cells of recombinant DNA? What target cells are to be treated *ex vivo* and returned to the patient? How will the cells be characterized before and after treatment? What is the theoretical and practical basis for assuming that only the target cells will incorporate the DNA?

II-B-2-a-(2). Is the delivery system efficient? What percentage of the target cells contain the added DNA?

II-B-2-a-(3). How is the structure of the added DNA sequences monitored and what is the sensitivity of the analysis? Is the added DNA extrachromosomal or integrated? Is the added DNA unrearranged?

II-B-2-a-(4). How many copies are present per cell? How stable is the added DNA both in terms of its continued presence and its structural stability?

II-B-2-b. Gene Transfer and Expression

II-B-2-b-(1). What animal and cultured cell models were used in laboratory studies to assess the *in vivo* and *in vitro* efficacy of the gene transfer system? In what ways are these models similar to and different from the proposed human treatment?

II-B-2-b-(2). What is the minimal level of gene transfer and/or expression that is estimated to be necessary for the gene transfer protocol to be successful in humans? How was this level determined?

II-B-2-b-(3). Explain in detail all results from animal and cultured cell model experiments which assess the effectiveness of the delivery system in achieving the minimally required level of gene transfer and expression.

II-B-2-b-(4). To what extent is expression only from the desired gene (and not from the surrounding DNA)? To what extent does the insertion modify the expression of other genes?

II-B-2-b-(5). In what percentage of cells does expression from the added DNA occur? Is the product biologically active? What percentage of normal activity results from the inserted gene?

II-B-2-b-(6). Is the gene expressed in cells other than the target cells? If so, to what extent?

II-B-2-c. Retrovirus Delivery Systems

II-B-2-c-(1). What cell types have been infected with the retroviral vector preparation? Which cells, if any, produce infectious particles?

II-B-2-c-(2). How stable are the retroviral vector and the resulting provirus against loss, rearrangement, recombination, or mutation? What information is available on how much rearrangement or recombination with endogenous or other viral sequences is likely to occur in the patient's cells? What steps have been taken in designing the vector to minimize instability or variation? What laboratory studies have been performed to check for stability, and what is the sensitivity of the analyses?

II-B-2-c-(3). What laboratory evidence is available concerning potential harmful effects of the transfer (e.g., development of neoplasia, harmful mutations, regeneration of infectious particles, or immune responses)? What steps will be taken in designing the vector to minimize pathogenicity? What laboratory studies have been performed to check for pathogencity, and what is the sensitivity of the analyses?

II-B-2-c-(4). Is there evidence from animal studies that vector DNA has entered untreated cells, particularly germ-line cells? What is the sensitivity of these analyses?

II-B-2-c-(5). Has a protocol similar to the one proposed for a clinical trial been conducted in non-human primates and/or other animals? What were the results? Specifically, is there any evidence that the retroviral vector has recombined with any endogenous or other viral sequences in the animals?

II-B-2-d. Non-Retrovirus Delivery/Expression Systems

If a non-retorviral delivery system is used, what animal studies have been conducted to determine if there are pathological or other undesirable consequences of the protocol (including insertion of DNA into cells other than those treated, particularly germ-line cells)? How long have the animals been studied after treatment? What safety studies have been conducted? (Include data about the level of sensitivity of such assays.)

II-B-3. Clinical Procedures, Including Patient Monitoring

Describe the treatment that will be administered to patients and the diagnostic methods that will be used to monitor the success or failure of the treatment. If previous clinical studies using similar methods have been performed by yourself or others, indicate their relevance to the proposed study. Specifically:

II-B-3-a. Will cells (e.g., bone marrow cells) be removed from patients and treated *ex vivo*? If so, describe the type, number, and intervals at which these cells will be removed.

II-B-3-b. Will patients be treated to eliminate or reduce the number of cells containing malfunctioning genes (e.g., through radiation or chemotherapy)?

II-B-3-c. What treated cells (or vector/DNA combination) will be given to patients? How will the treated cells be administered? What volume of cells will be used? Will there be single or multiple treatments? If so, over what period of time?

II-B-3-d. How will it be determined that new gene sequences have been inserted into the patient's cells and if these sequences are being expressed? Are these cells limited to the intended target cell populations? How sensitive are these analyses?

II-B-3-e. What studies will be conducted to assess the presence and effects of the contaminants?

II-B-3-f. What are the clinical endpoints of the study? Are there objectives and quantitative measurements to assess the natural history of the disease? Will such measurements be used in patient follow-up? How will patients be monitored to assess specific effects of the treatment on the disease? What is the sensitivity of the analyses? How frequently will follow-up studies be conducted? How long will patient follow-up continue?

II-B-3-g. What are the major beneficial and adverse effects of treatment that you anticipate? What measures will be taken in an attempt to control or reverse these adverse effects if they occur? Compare the probability and magnitude of deleterious consequences from the disease if recombinant DNA transfer is not used.

II-B-3-h. If a treated patient dies, what special post-mortem studies will be performed?

II-B-4. Public Health Considerations

Describe any potential benefits and hazards of the proposed therapy to persons other than the patients being treated. Specifically:

II-B-4-a. On what basis are potential public health benefits or hazards postulated?

II-B-4-b. Is there a significant possibility that the added DNA will spread from the patient to other persons or to the environment?

II-B-4-c. What precautions will be taken against such spread (e.g., patients sharing a room, health-care workers, or family members)?

II-B-4-d. What measures will be undertaken to mitigate the risks, if any, to public health?

II-B-4-e. In light of possible risks to offspring, including vertical transmission, will birth control measures be recommended to patients? Are such concerns applicable to health care personnel?

II-B-5. Qualifications of Investigators and Adequacy of Laboratory and Clinical Facilities

Indicate the relevant training and experience of the personnel who will be involved in the preclinical studies and clinical administration of recombinant DNA. Describe the laboratory and clinical facilities where the proposed study will be performed. Specifically:

II-B-5-a. What professional personnel (medical and nonmedical) will be involved in the proposed study and what is their relevant expertise? Provide a two-page curriculum vitae for each key professional person in biographical sketch format (see Appendix M-I, *Submission Requirements—Human Gene Transfer Proposals*).

II-B-5-b. At what hospital or clinic will the treatment be given? Which facilities of the hospital or clinic will be especially important for the proposed study? Will patients occupy regular hospital beds or clinical research center beds? Where will patients reside during the follow-up period? What special arrangements will be made for the comfort and consideration of the patients? Will the research institution designate an ombudsman, patient care representative, or other individual to help protect the rights and welfare of the patient?

II-C. Selection of the Patients

Estimate the number of patients to be involved in the proposed study. Describe recruitment procedures and patient eligibility requirements, paying particular attention to whether these procedures and requirements are fair and equitable. Specifically:

II-C-1. How many patients do you plan to involve in the proposed study?

II-C-2. How many eligible patients do you anticipate being able to identify each year?

II-C-3. What recruitment procedures do you plan to use?

II-C-4. What selection criteria do you plan to employ? What are the exclusion and inclusion criteria for the study?

II-C-5. How will patients be selected if it is not possible to include all who desire to participate?

III. Informed Consent

In accordance with the Protection of Human Subjects (45 CFR Part 46), investigators should indicate how subjects will be informed about the proposed study and the manner in which their consent will be solicited. They should indicate how the Informed Consent document makes clear the special requirements of gene transfer research. If a proposal involves children, special attention should be paid to the Protection of Human Subjects (45 CFR Part 46), Subpart D, Additional Protections for Children Involved as Subjects in Research.

III-A. Communication About the Study to Potential Participants

III-A-1. Which members of the research group and/or institution will be responsible for contacting potential participants and for describing the study to them? What procedures will be used to avoid possible conflicts of interest if the investigator is also providing medical care to potential subjects?

III-A-2. How will the major points covered in Appendix M-II, *Description of Proposal*, be disclosed to potential participants and/or their parents or guardians in language that is understandable to them?

III-A-3. What is the length of time that potential participants will have to make a decision about their participation in the study?

III-A-4. If the study involves pediatric or mentally handicapped subjects, how will the assent of each person be obtained?

III-B. Informed Consent Document

Investigators submitting human gene transfer proposals must include the Informed Consent document as approved by the local Institutional Review Board. A separate Informed Consent document should be used for the gene transfer portion of a research project when gene transfer is used as an adjunct in the study of another technique, e.g., when a gene is used as a "marker" or to enhance the power of immunotherapy for cancer.

Because of the relative novelty of the procedures that are used, the potentially irreversible consequences of the procedures performed, and the fact that many of the potential risks remain undefined, the Informed Consent document should include the following specific information in addition to any requirements of the DHHS regulations for the Protection of Human Subjects (45 CFR 46). Indicate if each of the specified items appears in the Informed Consent document or, if not included in the Informed Consent document, how those items will be presented to potential subjects. Include an explanation if any of the following items are omitted from the consent process or the Informed Consent document.

III-B-1. General Requirements of Human Subjects Research

III-B-1-a. Description/Purpose of the Study

The subjects should be provided with a detailed explanation in non-technical language of the purpose of the study and the procedures associated with the conduct of the proposed study, including a description of the gene transfer component.

III-B-1-b. Alternatives

The Informed Consent document should indicate the availability of therapies and the possibility of other investigational interventions and approaches.

III-B-1-c. Voluntary Participation

The subjects should be informed that participation in the study is voluntary and that failure to participate in the study or withdrawal of consent will not result in any penalty or loss of benefits to which the subjects are otherwise entitled.

III-B-1-d. Benefits

The subjects should be provided with an accurate description of the possible benefits, if any, of participating in the proposed study. For studies that are not reasonably expected to provide a therapeutic benefit to subjects, the Informed Consent document should clearly state that no direct clinical benefit to subjects is expected to occur as a result of participation in the study, although knowledge may be gained that may benefit others.

III-B-1-e. Possible Risks, Discomforts, and Side Effects

There should be clear itemization in the Informed Consent document of types of adverse experiences, their relative severity, and their expected frequencies. For consistency, the following definitions are suggested: side effects that are listed as mild should be ones which do not require a therapeutic intervention; moderate side effects require an intervention; and severe side effects are potentially fatal or life-threatening, disabling, or require prolonged hospitalization.

If verbal descriptors (e.g., "rare," "uncommon," or "frequent") are used to express quantitative information regarding risk, these terms should be explained.

The Informed Consent document should provide information regarding the approximate number of people who have previously received the genetic material under study. It is necessary to warn potential subjects that, for genetic materials previously used in relatively few or no humans, unforeseen risks are possible, including ones that could be severe.

The Informed Consent document should indicate any possible adverse medical consequences that may occur if the subjects withdraw from the study once the study has started.

III-B-1-f. Costs

The subjects should be provided with specific information about any financial costs associated with their participation in the protocol and in the long-term follow-up to the protocol that are not covered by the investigators or the institution involved.

Subjects should be provided an explanation about the extent to which they will be responsible for any costs for medical treatment required as a result of research-related injury.

III-B-2. Specific Requirements of Gene Transfer Research
III-B-2-a. Reproductive Considerations

To avoid the possibility that any of the reagents employed in the gene transfer research could cause harm to a fetus/child, subjects should be given information concerning possible risks and the need for contraception by males and females during the active phase of the study. The period of time for the use of contraception should be specified.

The inclusion of pregnant or lactating women should be addressed.

III-B-2-b. Long-Term Follow-Up

To permit evaluation of long-term safety and efficacy of gene transfer, the prospective subjects should be informed that they are expected to cooperate in long-term follow-up that extends beyond the active phase of the study. The Informed Consent document should include a list of persons who can be contacted in the event that questions arise during the follow-up period. The investigator should request that subjects continue to provide a current address and telephone number.

The subjects should be informed that any significant findings resulting from the study will be made known in a timely manner to them and/or their parent or guardian including new information about the experimental procedure, the harms and benefits experienced by other individuals involved in the study, and any long-term effects that have been observed.

III-B-2-c. Request for Autopsy

To obtain vital information about the safety and efficacy of gene transfer, subjects should be informed that at the time of death, no matter what the cause, permission for an autopsy will be requested of their families. Subjects should be asked to advise their families of the request and of its scientific and medical importance.

III-B-2-d. Interest of the Media and Others in the Research

To alert subjects that others may have an interest in the innovative character of the protocol and in the status of the treated subjects, the subjects should be informed of the following: (i) that the institution and investigators will make efforts to provide protection from the media in an effort to protect the participants' privacy, and (ii) that representatives of applicable Federal agencies (e.g., the National Institutes of Health and the Food and Drug Administration), representatives of collaborating institutions, vector suppliers, etc., will have access to the subjects' medical records.

IV. Privacy and Confidentiality

Indicate what measures will be taken to protect the privacy of patients and their families as well as to maintain the confidentiality of research data.

IV-A. What provisions will be made to honor the wishes of individual patients (and the parents or guardians of pediatric or mentally handicapped patients) as to whether, when, or how the identity of patients is publicly disclosed?

IV-B. What provisions will be made to maintain the confidentiality of research data, at least in cases where data could be linked to individual patients?

V. Special Issues

Although the following issues are beyond the normal purview of local institutional Review Boards, investigators should respond to the following questions:

V-A. What steps will be taken, consistent with Appendix M-IV *Privacy and Confidentiality*, to ensure that accurate and appropriate information is made available to the public with respect to such public concerns as may arise from the proposed study?

V-B. Do you or your funding sources intend to protect under patent or trade secret laws either the products or the procedures developed in the proposed study? If so, what steps will be taken to permit as full communication as possible among investigators and clinicians concerning research methods and results?

VI. RAC Review—Human Gene Transfer Protocols

VI-A. Categories of Human Gene Transfer Experiments that Require RAC Review

Factors that may contribute to the necessity for RAC review include, but are not limited to: (i) new vectors/new gene delivery systems, (ii) new diseases, (iii) unique applications of gene transfer, and (iv) other issues considered to require further public discussion. Whenever possible, investigators will be notified within 15 working days following receipt of the submission whether RAC review will be required. In the event that RAC review is deemed necessary by the NIH and FDA, the proposal will be forwarded to the RAC primary reviewers for evaluation. In order to maintain public access to information regarding human gene transfer protocols, NIH/ORDA will maintain the documentation described in Appendices M-I through M-V (including protocols that are not reviewed by the RAC).

VI-B. RAC Primary Reviewers' Written Comments

In the event that NIH/ORDA or the FDA recommend RAC review of the submitted proposal, the documentation described in Appendices M-I through M-V will be forwarded to the RAC primary reviewers for evaluation.

The RAC primary reviewers shall provide written comments on the proposal to NIH/ORDA. The RAC primary reviewers' comments should include the following:

VI-B-1. Emphasize the issues related to gene marking, gene transfer, or gene therapy.

VI-B-2. State explicitly whether Appendices M-I through M-V have been addressed satisfactorily.

VI-B-3. Examine the scientific rationale, scientific context (relative to other proposals reviewed by the RAC), whether the preliminary *in vitro* and *in vivo* data were obtained in appropriate models and are sufficient, and whether questions related to safety, efficacy, and social/ethical context have been resolved.

VI-B-4. Whenever possible, criticisms of Informed Consent documents should include written alternatives for suggested revisions for the RAC to consider.

VI-B-5. Primary reviews should state whether the proposal is: (i) acceptable as written, (ii) expected to be acceptable with specific revisions or after satisfactory responses to specific questions raised on review, or (iii) unacceptable in its present form.

VI-C. Investigator's Written Responses to RAC Primary Reviewers

VI-C-1. Written responses (including critical data in response to RAC primary reviewers' written comments) shall be submitted to NIH/ORDA greater than or equal to 2 weeks following receipt of the review.

VI-D. Oral Responses to the RAC

Investigators shall limit their oral responses to the RAC only to those questions that are raised during the meeting. Investigators are strongly discouraged from presenting critical data during their oral presentations that was not submitted greater than or equal to 2 weeks in advance of the RAC meeting at which it is reviewed.

VI-E. RAC Recommendations to the NIH Director

The RAC will recommend approval or disapproval of the reviewed proposal to the NIH Director. In the event that a proposal is contingently approved by the RAC, the RAC prefers that the conditions be satisfactorily met before the RAC's recommendation for approval is submitted to the NIH Director. The NIH Director's decision on the submitted proposal will be transmitted to the FDA Commissioner and considered as a *Major Action* by the NIH Director.

VII. Categories of Human Gene Transfer Experiments that May Be Exempt from RAC Review

A proposal submitted under one of the following categories may be considered exempt from RAC review unless otherwise determined by NIH/ORDA and the FDA on a case-by-case basis (see Appendix M-VI-A, *Categories of Human Gene Transfer Experiments that Require RAC Review*).

Note: In the event that the submitted proposal is determined to be exempt from RAC review, the documentation described in Appendices M-I through M-V will be maintained by NIH/ORDA for compliance with semiannual data reporting and adverse event reporting requirements (see Appendix M-VIII, *Reporting Requirements—Human Gene Transfer Protocols*). Any subsequent modifications to proposals that were not reviewed by the RAC must be submitted to NIH/ORDA in order to facilitate data reporting requirements.

VII-A. Vaccines

This category includes recombinant DNA vaccines not otherwise exempt from RAC review (see Appendix M-IX-A, *Footnotes of Appendix M*, for exempt vaccines).

VII-B. Lethally Irradiated Tumor Cells/No Replication-Competent Virus

This category includes experiments involving lethally irradiated tumor cells and: (1) vector constructs that have previously been approved by the RAC (or with the incorporation of minor modifications), or (2) a different tumor cell target.

VII-C. New Site/Original Investigator

This category includes the following: (1) initiation of a protocol at an additional site other than the site that was originally approved by the RAC, and (2) the investigator at the new site is the same as the investigator approved for the original study.

VII-D. New Site/New Investigator

This category includes the following: (1) initiation of a protocol at an additional site other than the site that was originally approved by the RAC, and (2) the investigator at the new site is different than the investigator approved for the original site.

VII-E. "Umbrella" Protocols

This category includes initiation of a RAC-approved protocol at more than one additional site (the Principal Investigator may be the same or different from the Principal Investigator approved for the original site).

VII-F. Modifications Related to Gene Transfer

This category includes experiments involving a modification to the clinical protocol that is not related to the gene transfer portion of study.

VII-G. Gene Marking Protocols

This category includes human gene marking experiments involving vector constructs that have previously been approved by the RAC and: (1) minor modifications to the vector constructs, or (2) a different tumor cell target.

VIII. Reporting Requirements—Human Gene Transfer Protocols

VIII-A. Semiannual Data Reporting

Investigators who have received approval from the FDA to initiate a human gene transfer protocol (whether or not it has been reviewed by the RAC) shall be required to comply with the semiannual data reporting requirements. Semi-annual Data Report forms will be forwarded by NIH/ORDA to investigators. Data submitted in these reports will be evaluated by the RAC, NIH/ORDA, and the FDA and reviewed by the RAC at its next regularly scheduled meeting.

VIII-B. Adverse Event Reporting

Investigators who have received approval from the FDA to initiate a human gene transfer protocol (whether or not it has been reviewed by the RAC) must report any serious adverse event immediately to the local IRB, IBC, NIH Office for Protection from Research Risks, NIH/ORDA, and FDA, followed by the submission of a written report filed with each group. Reports submitted to NIH/ORDA shall be sent to the Office of Recombinant DNA Activities, National Institutes of

Health, 6006 Executive Boulevard, Suite 323, Bethesda, Maryland 20892-7052, (301) 496-9838.

IX. Footnotes of Appendix M

IX-A. Human studies in which the induction or enhancement of an immune response to a vector-encoded microbial immunogen is the major goal, such an immune response has been demonstrated in model systems, and the persistence of the vector-encoded immunogen is not expected, may be initiated without RAC review if approved by another Federal agency.

Appendix E:
Background Information on
Homologous Recombination

Targeted Gene Replacement

Mario R. Capecchi

Every cell of our bodies has within its nucleus an instruction manual that specifies its function. Although each cell carries the same manual, different cell types, such as liver or skin, use different parts of this manual to detail their unique functions. Perhaps most remarkable, the manual contains the information that allows a one-cell embryo, the fertilized egg, to become a fetus and then a newborn child. As the child matures physically and intellectually, he or she is still using the information within the instruction manual. We are each unique, and the manual is slightly different for each of us; it specifies most of the physical and many of the behavioral characteristics that distinguish us as individuals.

This extraordinary manual, otherwise known as the genome, is written in the form of nucleotides, four of which constitute the entire alphabet—adenylate (*A*), cytidylate (*C*), guanylate (*G*) and thymidylate (*T*). It is the precise sequence of the nucleotides in DNA that conveys information, much as the sequence of letters in a word conveys meaning. During each cell division, the entire manual is replicated, and a copy is handed down from the mother cell to each of its two daughters. In humans and mice, the manuals each contain three billion nucleotides. If the letters representing the nucleotides were written down in order so that a page carried 3,000 characters, the manual would occupy 1,000 volumes, each consist-

Source: *Scientific American* 270(3): 52–59; March 1994. Reprinted by permission of Scientific American, Inc. Illustrations omitted.

ing of 1,000 pages. Thus, a very complex manual is required to orchestrate the creation of a human or mouse from a fertilized egg.

Recently my colleagues at the University of Utah and I developed the technology for specifically changing a letter, a sentence or several paragraphs in the instruction manual within every cell of a living mouse. By rewriting parts of the manual and evaluating the consequences of the altered instructions on the development or the postdevelopmental functioning of the mouse, we can gain insight into the program that governs these processes.

The functional units within the instruction manual are genes. We specifically change the nucleotide sequence of a chosen gene and thereby alter its function. For instance, if we suspected a particular gene were involved in brain development, we could generate mouse embryos in which the normal gene was "knocked out"—that is, completely inactivated. If this inactivation caused newborn mice to have a malformed cerebellum, we would know that the gene in question was essential to forming that part of the brain. The process by which specified changes are introduced into the nucleotide sequence of a chosen gene is termed gene targeting.

Much of what is learned from gene-targeting experiments in mice should benefit humans, because an estimated 99 percent or more of the genes in mice and humans are the same and serve quite similar purposes. Application of the technology in mice is already clarifying not only the steps by which human embryonic development occurs but also the ways in which our immune system is formed and used to fight infection. Gene targeting should also go far toward explaining such mysteries as how the human brain operates and how defects in genes give rise to disease. In the latter effort the technique is being used to produce mouse models of human disorders—among them, cystic fibrosis, cancer and atherosclerosis.

Excitement over gene targeting stems from another source as well. It promises to expand on the knowledge generated by the genome project. This large-scale undertaking aims to determine the nucleotide sequence of every gene in the mouse and human genomes (approximately 200,000 genes in each). Currently we know the functions of only a minute percentage of the genes in either species. The nucleotide sequence of a gene specifies the amino acids that must be strung together to make a particular protein. (Proteins carry out most of the activities in cells.) The amino acid sequence of a protein yields important clues to its roles in cells, such as whether it serves as an enzyme, a structural component of the cell or a signaling molecule. But the sequence alone is not sufficient to reveal the particular tasks performed by the protein during the life of the animal. In contrast, gene targeting can provide this information and thereby move our understanding of the functions of genes and their proteins to a much deeper level.

Gene targeting offers investigators a new way to do mammalian genetics—that is, to determine how genes mediate various biological processes. This technique was needed because the classical methods of genetics, which have been highly successful in analyzing biological processes in simpler organisms, were not readily adaptable to organisms as complex as mammals.

If geneticists want to learn, for example, how single-cell organisms, such as bacteria or yeast, replicate their DNA, they can expose a billion or more individuals to a DNA-damaging chemical (a mutagen). By choosing the right dosage of mutagen, they can ensure that each individual in that population carries a mutation in one or more genes. From this population of mutagenized bacteria or yeast, the geneticists can identify individuals not capable of replicating their DNA. The use of such a large mutagenized population makes it likely that separate individuals will be found with mutations in each of the genes required for DNA replication. (For a process as complicated as duplicating the bacterial or yeast genome, more than 100 genes are involved.) Once the individual genes are identified, their specific role in DNA replication, such as which genes control the decision to copy the DNA and which control the accuracy and rate of copying, can be determined.

Similar approaches have been applied to multicellular organisms, which are more complex. Two favorites of geneticists are *Caenorhabditis elegans*, a tiny, soil-dwelling worm, and *Drosophila melanogaster*, a common fruit fly. But even in these relatively simple forms of multicellular organisms, identifying all the genes involved in a specific biological process is more demanding.

A number of factors contribute to this increased difficulty. One is the size of the genome. The genome of the bacterium *Escherichia coli* includes only 3,000 genes, whereas that of *D. melanogaster* contains at least 20,000 genes; the mouse genome contains 10 times that number. With added genes comes added complexity, because the genes form more intricate, interacting networks. Tracing the effect of any one gene in such an involved network is a formidable task.

Moreover, the larger size of multicellular organisms places practical limits on the number of individuals that can be included in a mutagenesis experiment. It is fairly simple and inexpensive to search for specific kinds of mutants among more than a billion mutagenized bacteria or yeast. In contrast, screening even 100,000 mutagenized fruit flies would constitute a large experiment. By comparison, the practical limits on screening mice for a particular mutation would be reached at about 1,000 animals.

The logistical difficulties of identifying and studying genes in multicellular organisms are further increased by the fact that most are diploid—their cells carry two copies of most genes, one inherited from the father and a second from the mother. For survival purposes, having two copies of most genes is valuable. If one copy acquires a harmful mutation, the other copy can usually compensate, so that no serious consequences result. Such redundancy, however, means that a mutation will elicit anatomical or physiological defects in the organism only if both copies of the gene are damaged. Investigators produce such individuals by mating parents who each carry the mutation in one copy of the gene. Approximately one fourth of the offspring of such matings will bear two defective copies of the gene. The need for matings introduces delays in the analysis.

Despite the challenges, the identification of selected mutations in whole animals is unquestionably the most informative way to begin clarifying and separating the steps by which biological processes are carried out. Furthermore, if we want to understand processes that occur only in complex organisms, such as the mounting of a sophisticated immune response, such analysis must be pursued in those organisms. For these reasons, geneticists interested in mammalian development, neural function, immune response, physiology and disease have turned to the mouse. From a geneticist's point of view, the mouse is an ideal mammal. It is small and prolific and serves as a remarkably good analogue for most human biological processes.

On the other hand, the breadth of genetic manipulations that can be carried out in mice has been extremely limited relative to the operations that are possible in simpler organisms. Because of the obstacles I have already described, it is not practical to apply classical techniques to mice. To identify mutagenized mice carrying defects in the genes involved in some process of interest, researchers would have to screen 10,000 to 100,000 mice at a prohibitive cost. Instead mouse geneticists have historically studied mutant animals that arose spontaneously within their colonies. As a result of the keen observation and perseverance by such workers, the collection of existing mouse mutants is surprisingly large and is an invaluable resource for continued research.

Yet even these hard-won animals have drawbacks. The existing collection of mutant mice does not harbor a random sampling of mutations in the mouse genome. Rather it contains a disproportionate number of mutations that result in readily observable abnormalities in physiology or behavior. In consequence, many mutations that affect coat color are present in this collection, whereas mutations that affect early development are underrepresented (since they often result in the undetected death of the embryo).

Further, the task of isolating the genes responsible for overt defects in mutant mice is very labor intensive, often taking years of concerted effort. Workers can deduce many steps involved in biological phenomena without ever finding the genes involved. But without isolating those genes, they cannot make progress at the molecular level. Notably, they cannot determine the nature of the proteins encoded by the mutated genes, nor can they identify the cells in which the genes are active.

Gene targeting allows investigators to circumvent such difficulties. Investigators now choose which gene to alter. They also have virtually complete control over how that gene is modified, so that the mutation can be tailor-made to address precise questions about the functions of the gene. The criteria for selecting which gene to mutate can be based on knowledge obtained from research on mice or other species. For example, it is now relatively straightforward to isolate a series of genes that are active in the newly forming mouse heart; gene targeting would then permit determining the role of each of those genes in heart development. Alternatively, we can ascertain whether a set of genes known to be involved in guiding the paths taken by developing neurons in *D. melanogaster* exist and serve a similar function in the mouse.

An initial approach often involves knocking out a gene in order to evaluate the consequences to the organism of not having the gene product. The consequences may be complex and may affect multiple pathways. Further insight into the gene's function can be obtained by introducing more subtle, defined mutations, which may affect only one of its multiple roles. Soon geneticists should be able to place genes under control of a switch. Such switches will allow researchers to turn a gene on and off during the embryonic or postnatal development of the mouse. For example, a hypothetical gene could be responsible for the creation and proper operation of a set of nerve cells. Knocking out the gene would result in the absence of those neurons during formation of the brain and preclude assessing the gene's activity in the adult. If the gene were under control of a switch, however, the switch could be left on during development, and the neurons would be formed. In the adult the switch could then be turned off, enabling workers to evaluate the function of this gene in adult neurons.

Development of gene-targeting technology has evolved over the past 15 years. In the late 1970s I was experimenting with using extremely small glass needles to inject DNA directly into the nuclei of mammalian cells. The needles were controlled by hydraulically driven micromanipulators and directed into nuclei with the aid of a high-powered microscope. The procedure turned out to be extremely efficient. One in three to five cells received the DNA in a functional form and went on to divide and stably pass that DNA on to its daughter cells.

When I followed the fate of these DNA molecules in cells, a surprising phenomenon captured my attention. Although the newly introduced DNA molecules were randomly inserted into one of the recipient cell's chromosomes, more than one molecule could be inserted at that site, and all of them were in the same orientation. Just as words in any language have an orientation (in English we read words from left to right), so, too, do DNA molecules. Apparently, before cells performed random insertion, some mechanism in the cell nucleus stitched virtually all the introduced DNA molecules together in the same orientation.

We went on to demonstrate that cells used a process called homologous recombination to achieve such linkages. Homologous recombination works only on DNA molecules with the same nucleotide sequence. Such molecules line up next to each other. Then both molecules are cut and are joined to each other at the cut ends. The joining is accomplished with such precision that the nucleotide sequences at the points of linkage are not altered.

This unexpected observation implied that all mouse cells, and presumably all mammalian cells, had the machinery to perform homologous recombination. At the time, there was no reason to suspect that somatic cells (those not involved in sexual reproduction) would have this machinery. Further, we knew the machinery was fairly efficient because we could microinject more than 100 DNA molecules of the same sequence, and the cell would stitch them all together in the same orientation. I realized immediately that if we could harness this machinery to carry out homologous recombination between a newly introduced DNA molecule of our choice and the same DNA sequence in a cell's chromosome, we would have the ability to rewrite the cell's instruction manual at will.

Excited by this prospect, in 1980 I requested funding from the government to test the feasibility of gene targeting. To my disappointment, the scientists who reviewed the grant proposal rejected it. In their view, the probability that the newly introduced DNA sequence would ever find its matching sequence within the 1,000 volumes of the genetic instruction manual seemed vanishingly small.

Despite the rejection, I decided to forge ahead using funds I was receiving for another project. It was a gamble. Had the experiments failed, I would have had little meaningful data to submit at grant renewal time. Fortunately, the experiments worked. By 1984, when we again asked for funds to pursue the research, we had ample evidence that gene targeting was in fact feasible in cells. Many of the same scientists who had reviewed the original grant proposal now demonstrated a sense of humor. The critique of the new proposal opened with the statement, "We are glad that you didn't follow our advice."

How is gene targeting in cells accomplished? The first step is to clone the gene of interest and propagate it in bacteria. This procedure provides a pure source of DNA containing the gene. Next, in a test tube, the nucleotide sequence of the gene is changed to meet the purpose of the experiment. The altered gene is referred to as the targeting vector.

The targeting vector is introduced into living cells by any of several means. Once within the cell nucleus, it forms a complex with proteins constituting the cell's machinery for homologous recombination. Aided by these proteins, it searches through all the sequences of the genome until it finds its counterpart (the target). If it indeed does find its target, it will line up next to that gene and replace it.

Regrettably, such targeted replacement occurs only in a small fraction of the treated cells. More often, the targeting vector inserts randomly at non-matching sites or fails to integrate at all. We must therefore sort through the cells to identify those in which targeting has succeeded. Approximately one in a million treated cells has the desired targeted replacement.

To greatly simplify the search for that cell, we make use of two "selectable markers," which are introduced into the targeting vector from the start. Inclusion of a "positive" selectable marker promotes survival and growth of cells that have incorporated the targeting vector, either at the target site or at a random location within the genome. Inclusion of the "negative" selectable marker helps to eliminate most of the cells that have incorporated the targeting vector at a random location.

The positive marker, usually a *neomycin-resistance* (*neo^r*) gene, is positioned so that it will be flanked by DNA also present in the target gene. The negative marker, typically the *thymidine kinase* (*tk*) gene from a herpes virus, is attached to one end of the targeting vector. . . . When homologous recombination occurs, the unchanged segments of the cloned gene, together with the *neo^r* gene sandwiched between them, replace the target sequence in the chromosome. But the *tk* gene, lying outside the zone of matching sequences, does not enter the chromosome and is degraded by the cell. In contrast, when cells randomly insert the targeting vector, they stitch the entire vector, complete with the *tk* gene, into the DNA. When no insertion occurs, the vector and both its markers are lost.

We do not have to examine the DNA directly to identify these different outcomes. Instead we grow the cells in a medium containing two drugs, an analogue of neomycin called G418 and the antiherpes drug ganciclovir. G418 kills cells that lack the protective *neo^r* gene in their chromosomes, namely, those that have failed to integrate vector DNA. But it allows cells that carry either random or targeted insertions to survive and grow. Concurrently the ganciclovir kills any cells that carry the herpes *tk* gene, namely, those that harbor a random insertion. In the end, virtually the only surviving cells are those bearing the targeted insertion (cells possessing the "positive selectable" *neo^r* gene and lacking the "negative selectable" *tk* gene).

By 1984 we had shown that it was possible to target specific genes in cultured mouse cells. We were then ready to extend the technology to alter the genome of living mice. To accomplish this aim, we used special cells developed in 1981 by Matthew H. Kaufman and Martin J. Evans of the University of Cambridge. These cells are embryo-derived stem (ES) cells. Such cells are obtained from an early mouse embryo. They can be cultured in petri dishes indefinitely, and they are pluripotent: capable of giving rise to all cell types.

In brief, by the procedure described earlier, we produce ES cells known to carry a targeted mutation in one copy of a chosen gene. Then we put the ES cells into early mouse embryos, which are allowed to develop to term. Some of the resulting mice, when mature, will produce sperm derived from the ES cells. By mating such mice to normal mice, we generate offspring that are heterozygous for the mutation—they carry the mutation in one of the two copies of the gene in every cell.

These heterozygotes will be healthy in most instances, because their second, undamaged copy of the gene will still be functioning properly. But mating of these heterozygotes to brothers or sisters bearing the same mutation yields homozygotes: animals carrying the targeted mutation in both copies of the gene. Such animals will display abnormalities that will reveal the normal functions of the target gene in all their tissues.

Of course, the procedure is more easily summarized than carried out. To actually do the work, we begin by injecting our modified ES cells into blastocyst-stage embryos, which have not yet become attached to the mother's uterus. Because we depend on coat color to indicate whether the procedure is going according to plan, we choose blastocysts that would normally develop into pups bearing a different coat color than is found in pups produced by the mouse strain from which the ES cells are obtained.

The stem cells are isolated from a brown mouse carrying two copies of the *agouti* gene. This gene, even when present in a single copy, produces brown coloring by causing yellow pigment to be laid down next to black pigment in the hair shaft. (Production of the pigments themselves is under the control of other genes.) Hence, we typically select blastocysts that would normally develop into black mice. (Mice acquire black coats when the *agouti* gene inherited from both parents is defective.) Then we allow the embryo, containing the modified ES cells, to grow to term in a surrogate mother.

If all goes well, the altered ES cells reproduce repeatedly during this time, passing complete copies of all their genes to their daughter cells. These cells mix with those of the embryo and contribute to the formation of most mouse tissues. As a result, the newborns are chimeras: they are composed of cells derived both frim the foreign ES cells and from the original embryo. We readily identify such chimeras by observing broad swatches of brown coloring in their otherwise black coats. If the animals bore no ES-derived cells, they would be completely black because of their lack of functional *agouti* genes.

By merely looking at the chimeras, though, we cannot determine whether the ES cells gave rise to germ cells, the vehicle through which the targeted mutation is passed to future generations. We find that out only when we move to the next stage: producing heterozygous mice harboring one copy of the mutation in all their cells. To generate such animals, we mate chimeric male mice to black female mice lacking the *agouti* gene. An offspring will be brown if the sperm that fertilized the egg was derived from ES cells (because all such sperm carry the *agouti* gene). An offspring will be black if the sperm derived from the original blastocyst cells (which lack functional *agouti* genes).

Consequently, when we see brown pups, we know that the genes carried by ES cells made their way to these offspring. We can then think about setting up matings between heterozygous siblings in order to produce mice with two defective copies of the target gene. First, though, we must discern which of the brown pups carry a copy of the mutated gene. This we do by examing their DNA directly for the targeted mutation. When matings are set up between heterozygous siblings, one in four of the offspring will have two defective copies of the gene. We pick out the homozygotes by again analyzing DNA directly, this time looking for the presence of two copies of the targeted mutation. These animals are then examined carefully for any anatomical, physiological or behavioral anomalies that can provide clues to the functions of the disrupted gene. The total procedure from cloning a gene to generating mice with a targeted mutation in that gene takes approximately one year.

Laboratories all around the world are now applying gene targeting in mice to study an array of biological problems. Since 1989, more than 250 strains carrying selected genetic defects have been produced. A few examples of the emerging findings should illustrate the kinds of insights these animals can provide.

In my own laboratory, we have been exploring the functions of homeotic, or *Hox*, genes. These genes serve as master switches ensuring that different parts of the body, such as the limbs, the organs, and parts of the head, form in the appropriate places and take on the correct shapes. Studies of homeotic genes in *Drosophila* have yielded important clues to their activities [see "The Molecular Architects of Body Design," by William McGinnis and Michael Kuziora; SCIENTIFIC AMERICAN, February (1994)]. Yet many questions remain. For instance, *D. melanogaster* has only eight *Hox* genes, whereas mice and humans each have 38. Presumably, expansion of the *Hox* family played a critical part in the evolutionary progression from invertebrates to vertebrates, supplying extra machinery needed for a more complex body. Precisely what do all 38 genes do?

Before gene targeting became available, there was no way to answer these questions, because no one had found mice or humans with mutations in any of the 38 *Hox* genes. My colleagues and I are now embarking on a systematic effort to establish the function of the individual *Hox* genes. Later we will attempt to identify how these genes form an interactive network to direct the formation of our bodies.

As part of this program, we have discovered that targeted disruption of the *HoxA-3* gene leads to multiple defects. Mice carrying two mutated copies of the gene die at birth from cardiovascular dysfunction brought on by incomplete development of the heart and the major blood vessels issuing from it. These mice are also born with aberrations in many other tissues, including the thymus and parathyroid (which are missing), the thyroid gland, the bone and cartilage of the lower head, and the connective tissue, muscle and cartilage of the throat.

These abnormalities are diverse but share one striking commonality: the affected tissues all descend from cells that were originally clustered in a narrow zone in the upper part of the developing embryo. The rudiments of the heart, for instance, are located in this region before the heart takes up its more posterior location in the chest. It seems, then, that the assignment of the *HoxA-3* gene is to oversee construction of many of the tissues and organs that originate in this narrow region.

Unexpectedly, the disorder produced by knocking out the mouse *HoxA-3* gene mimics that found in an inherited human disease known as DiGeorge syndrome. Chromosomal analysis of patients shows that the human *HoxA-3* gene is not the culprit; victims display genetic damage on a chromosome distinct from that housing *HoxA-3*. We now know, however, that the gene responsible for the syndrome acts by interfering either with activation of the *HoxA-3* gene or with the events set in motion by the *HoxA-3* gene. Also, a mouse model for the disease is now available and may eventually provide clues to treatment. This unanticipated benefit underscores once again the value of basic research: findings born of curiosity often lead to highly practical applications.

Like developmental biologists, immunologists have also benefited from gene targeting. They are now applying this technology to decipher the individual responsibilities of well over 50 genes that influence the development and operation of the body's two foremost classes of defensive cells—*B* and *T* lymphocytes.

Cancer researchers are excited by the technique as well. Often investigators know that mutations in a particular gene are common in one or more tumor types, but they do not know the normal role of the gene. Discovery of that role using our knockout technology can help to reveal how the mutant form of the gene contributes to malignancy.

The *p53* tumor suppressor gene offers a case in point. Tumor suppressor genes are ones whose inactivation contributes to the development or progression of cancer. Mutations in the *p53* gene are found in perhaps 80 percent of all human cancers, but until recently the precise responsibilities of the normal genes were obscure. The analysis of mice homozygous for a targeted disruption of *p53* indicated that *p53* probably acts as a watchdog that blocks healthy cells from dividing until they have repaired any damaged DNA that is present in the cell. Such damage often occurs in cells as a consequence of the frequent environmental insults to which we are subjected. The loss of functional *p53* genes eliminates this safeguard, allowing damaged DNA to be passed to daughter cells, where it participates in formation of cancers.

Many other diseases will be amenable to study by gene targeting. More than 5,000 human disorders have been attributed to genetic defects. As the genes and mutations for the disorders are identified, workers can create precisely the same mutations in mice. The mouse models, in turn, should make it possible to trace in detail the events leading from the malfunctioning of a gene to the manifestation of disease. A deeper understanding of the molecular pathology of the disease should permit the development of more effective therapies. Among the models now being constructed are mice with different mutations in the cystic fibrosis gene.

The study of atherosclerosis, a leading cause of strokes and heart attacks, is also beginning to involve gene targeting. In contrast to cystic fibrosis, atherosclerosis is not caused by mutations in a single gene. Defects in a number of genes combine with environmental factors to promote the buildup of plaque in arteries. Nevertheless, promising mouse models have been made by altering genes known to be involved in the processing of triglycerides and cholesterol. I also anticipate that mouse models for hypertension, another culprit in heart disease and stroke, will soon be developed, now that genes thought to participate in its development are being identified.

As understanding of the genetic contribution to disease increases, so will the desire to correct the defects by gene therapy. At the moment, the techniques used for gene therapy rely on random insertion of healthy genes into chromosomes, to compensate for the damaged version. But the inserted genes often do not function as effectively as they would if they occupied their assigned places on the chromosome. In principle, gene targeting can provide a solution to this problem. Yet, before it can be used to correct the defective gene in a patient's tissue, investigators may need to establish cultures of cells able to participate in formation of that tissue in adults. Such cells, which like the ES cells in our studies are termed stem cells, are known to be present in bone marrow, liver, lungs, skin, intestines and other tissues. But research into ways to isolate and culture these cells is still in its infancy.

Before the technical hurdles to broad application of our methods in gene therapy are surmounted, gene targeting will find common usage in the study of mammalian neurobiology. Already mice have been prepared with targeted mutations that alter their ability to learn. As increasing numbers of neural-specific genes are identified, the pace of this research will surely intensify.

We can anticipate continued improvements in gene-targeting technology, but it has already created opportunities to manipulate the mammalian genome in ways that were unimaginable even a few years ago. To significantly aid in deciphering the mechanisms underlying such complex processes as development or learning in mammals, researchers will have to call on every bit of their available ingenuity, carefully deciding which genes to alter and modifying those genes in ways that will bring forth informative answers. Gene targeting opens a broad range of possibilities for genetic manipulations, the limitations of which will be set only by the creative limits of our collective imagination.

Index

WANNA BET?

Also by Don Wade

WANNA BET?

The Greatest True Stories About Gambling on Golf,
from Titanic Thompson to Tiger Woods

DON WADE

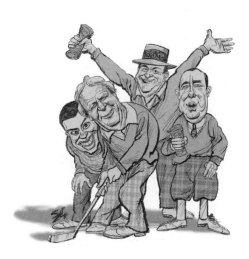

THUNDER'S MOUTH PRESS
NEW YORK

WANNA BET?
The Greatest True Stories About Gambling on Golf,
from Titanic Thompson to Tiger Woods

Copyright © 2005 by Don Wade
Illustrations © 2005 by Paul Szep

AVALON
publishing group incorporated

Published by
Thunder's Mouth Press
An Imprint of Avalon Publishing Group
245 West 17th Street, 11th Floor
New York, NY 10011

First printing November 2005

Library of Congress Cataloging-in-Publication Data is available.

ISBN: 1-56025-705-9
ISBN 13: 978-1-56025-705-9

9 8 7 6 5 4 3 2 1

Book design by Maria E. Torres
Printed in the United States
Distributed by Publishers Group West

To my dad—

The mayor of West Concord,
The King of Scrambles,
A great role model,
And an even better man

Thanks, Dad. This one's for you.

CONTENTS

ACKNOWLEDGMENTS

Over the years, I've come to appreciate just how much writing a book is a collaborative effort. For that reason, I want to thank some important people who helped make this book possible.

First, thanks to my editor at Avalon Publishing Group, Jofie Ferrari-Adler. This book was his idea and he's been a delight to work with—patient, supportive, and good-natured. I hope this is just the first of many books we do together.

Next up is Tara Mark, who handled this project as my agent at RLR. She, too, has been a wealth of encouragement and good advice when it comes to navigating the murky waters of publishing. Both she and her advice are much appreciated.

Then there is my old friend Paul Szep, who did the

illustrations. He and I go back a long way and I have admired his work since his first years at the *Boston Globe*, where he won two Pulitzers for his brilliance in comforting the afflicted and afflicting the comfortable. Now, if he could just find one good golf swing and stick with it . . . Thanks, Szeppy.

Then there are all my friends, who contributed so many stories and so much support.

Finally, thanks to Julia, Ben, Darcy, and Andy for their understanding, help, and love. No one could ask for more.

PREFACE

By a happy accident of both birth and fate, I have been around the game of golf virtually all my life.

My mother had two brothers who were golf professionals and a third brother who sold golf equipment for MacGregor. As a result, there were always clubs and balls around the house.

I grew up in Concord, Massachusetts, in a house that was just down the road from the Concord Country Club, a wonderful old club that dates back to the 1800s. Concord is the birthplace of democracy in America. I think Concord Country Club is probably the birthplace of the "nickel nassau." Everything I know and believe about golf gambling is rooted in my many happy years at Concord.

I started caddying when I was twelve years old. The

very first person I caddied for was a delightful old Yankee named Hope Chase. Mrs. Chase was a warm and funny woman and a very good player. However, on my first hole as a caddie, Mrs. Chase knocked her second shot into some thick grass bordering a pond, and, despite our best efforts, it was lost. I felt terrible and volunteered to buy her a new ball after the round.

"Don't worry about it, dear," she said. "I win more of these damned things than I can ever lose."

There were a lot of characters at Concord. One of my favorites was an old codger named Jack Codding, who had an uncanny knack for making holes-in-one. At that time, the company that distributed Drambuie—a Scottish liqueur that, when combined with Scotch whisky, produces the world's greatest cold-weather drink, a Rusty Nail—sponsored a sweepstakes. If you made a hole-in-one, you were eligible to enter. First prize was an all-expenses-paid trip to play the classic courses of Scotland.

Well, as luck would have it, Jack Codding won . . . but there was a hitch. If he accepted, the United States Golf Association would revoke his amateur status. As I recall, Mr. Codding thought it over, decided his chances of ever winning a tournament requiring that he be a certifiable amateur were nil, took the trip, and had a marvelous time.

When I look back on that time, I remember the caddie days, when we'd come to the course on Monday mornings and play all day for free. We'd have all sorts of little bets—greenies, sandies, barkies, Hogans, and Palmers. It seemed like every week somebody would come up with a new game or a new twist on an old one. I also remember that during the club championship, we'd bet on our favorite players. Mine was a guy named Bill O'Brien, a former Marine who looked like John Wayne, had a swing like Sam Snead's, and smoked Lucky Strikes that he lit with a Zippo. After he left the Marines, he became a banker, but I don't think his heart was ever really in it. His heart was in golf.

My first real introduction to the intricacies of gambling came in my senior year of high school, when I was working as an assistant in the golf shop. Johnny Devlin, who also worked in the shop, was a few years older than me and a very fine player. He went to the University of Florida at a time in Concord when going south to college meant going to Yale.

At any rate, that summer he arrived at the club with a brand-new set of Spalding Elite irons, which were beautiful clubs. As I looked at them, I noticed that the 6-iron seemed to have less loft than the 5-iron. In fact, the more I studied the irons, the more I was convinced that the lofts were all screwed up. When I mentioned this to Johnny, he just smiled. It turned out that when he'd ordered the clubs, he had Spalding deliberately mismark some of the numbers on the soles of the irons—the better to throw off any opponent who foolishly tried to go to school on his club selection.

This gambling business was tricky stuff, I was discovering.

In 1978, I went to work as an editor at *Golf Digest* and, happily, the first story I ever did was with Sam Snead. We struck up a wonderful friendship and I wound up working on all his stories for the magazine, as well as coauthoring a book with the Slammer. Along the way, we played a lot of golf and I heard a lot of stories. I developed the same sort of relationship with Amy Alcott, Tom Kite, and many others who I count as friends.

At that time, *Golf Digest* used to hold what were called "Pro Panel" meetings. These were usually three-day sessions attended by some of the greatest teachers in the game—Sam, Dr. Cary "Doc" Middlecoff, Paul Runyan, Bob Toski, Davis Love, Jr., Jim Flick, Peter Kostis, Chuck Cook, Jack Lumpkin, John Elliott, Dr. Bob Rotella, and many others. They were wonderful occasions, not least because of the stories that were told.

Many of them are in this book. I hope you enjoy them.

—Don Wade